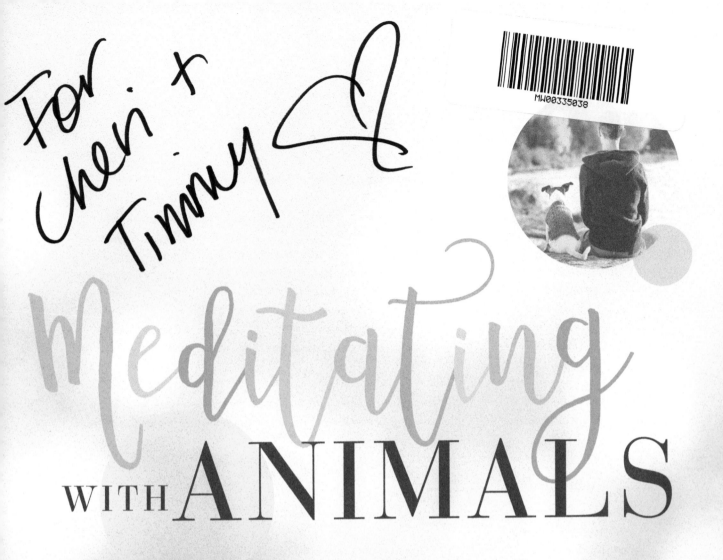

Meditating
WITH ANIMALS

HOW TO CREATE MORE CONSCIOUS CONNECTIONS WITH THE HEALERS AND TEACHERS AMONG US

Pamela

PAMELA ROBINS

Library of Congress Cataloging-in-Publication Data is available: 2016915490
ISBN 978-0-692-76855-6

Substantive editor and copy editor: Lindsay Humphreys
Proofreader: Christina Roth
Cover and interior designer: Domini Dragoone, www.dominidragoone.com
Front cover photo: © Lyss Nichole

Cold Canyon Press
www.MeditatingWithAnimals.com

9 8 7 6 5 4 3 2 1

Photo Credits: Pages iii, 16, 26, 36, 38, 41, 43, 44, 58, 59, 95, 119, 129, 138, 148, 149, 150, and 155 (top) © Pamela Robins. Pages 9, 64, 82, 154, 155 (bottom), and 158 © Mariana Schulze. Page 19 © Becke Corken. Page 57 © Alena Ozerova. Page 63 © Lisa Takada. Page 67 © Sylvain Hawawini. Page 75 © Colette Brooks. Page 99 © Jay Weiner photo of Ellie Laks, Founder of the Gentle Barn. Pages 114, 115, and 116 © Victoria Nodiff-Netanel, Founder Mini Therapy Horses. Page 117 © Steve Sullivan - Mini Therapy Horses. Page 123 © Molly McDonough. Page 132 © Tricia Meteer - Equinox Photo. The following photos were sourced from 123RF.com: (page) i © DameDeeso, iv © Jaromír Chalabala, vi © Sergejs Rahunoks, 1 © Michal Bednarek, 3 © Aliaksei Lasevich, 6 © Susan Richey-Schmitz, 10-11 © Paul Higley, 12 © GVN, 15 © Jozef Klopacka, 20 © Nelik, 25 © Rashid Valitov, 28 © Wavebreak Media Ltd, 35 © Andrea Obzerova, 40 © Yulia Chupina, 46 © dmosreg, 53 © Deborah Kolb, 55 © Christin Gasner, 60 © DameDeeso, 68 © Ann Ems, 71 © Mona Makela, 72 (top) © Tom Baker, 76 © Mykola Kravchenko, 77 © Aleksandr Davydov, 84 © DameDeeso, 91 © Konstantin Tronin, 94 © Ysbrand Cosijn, 97 © Inga Makeyeva, 98 © Alexsandrs Tihinovs, 101 © VV Vita, 103 © Oleksii Leonov, 104 © Oleg Itki, 107 © Xalanx, 108 © Fabio Formaggio, 110 © Bernd Juergens, 113 © Ammentorp, 120 © Kongkit Chumtap, 126 © Nataliia Kelsheva, 131 © Nattawut Jaroenchai, 134 © Tibanna79, 136 © Belchonock, 139 © Pavel Ilyukhin, 140 © Ramona Smiers, 145 © Chadchai Rangubpai, 146 © Peter Hermes Furian. The following photos were sourced from iStock.com: (page) 22 © Pentium2, 32 © Svetikd, 50 © Bartosz Hadyniak, 72 (bottom) © Milos Stankovic, 81 © Tatiana Morozova, 88 © Wundervisuals, 133 © Daniel Bendjy.

*I would like to dedicate
this work to all the
animals who have been an
integral part of my life
and who showed me what
unconditional love is beyond
a shadow of a doubt.*

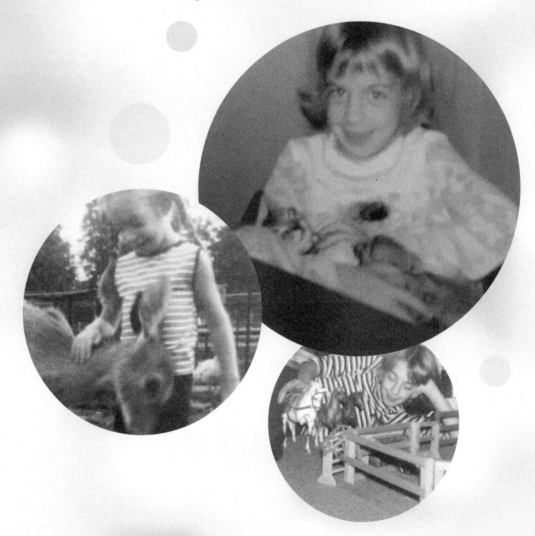

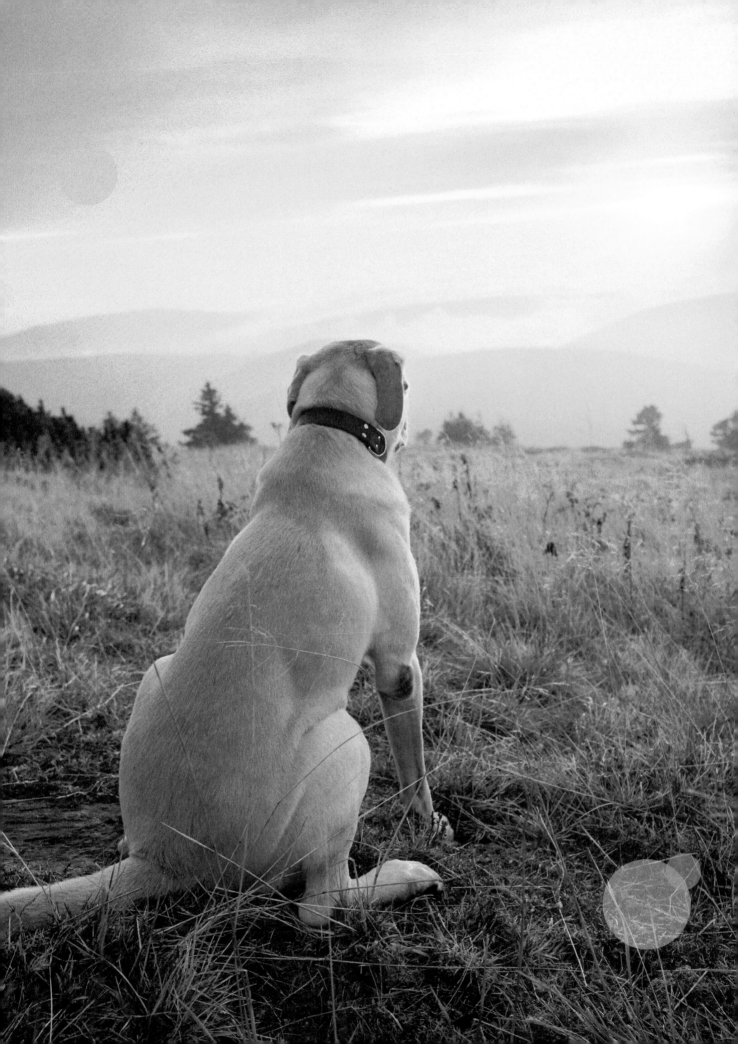

Near this spot
are deposited the remains
of one who possessed
Beauty without *Vanity*

Strength without Insolence

Courage without *Ferocity*

And all the *Virtues* of
Man without his Vices.

—LORD BYRON
(written in honor of his dog, Boatswain)

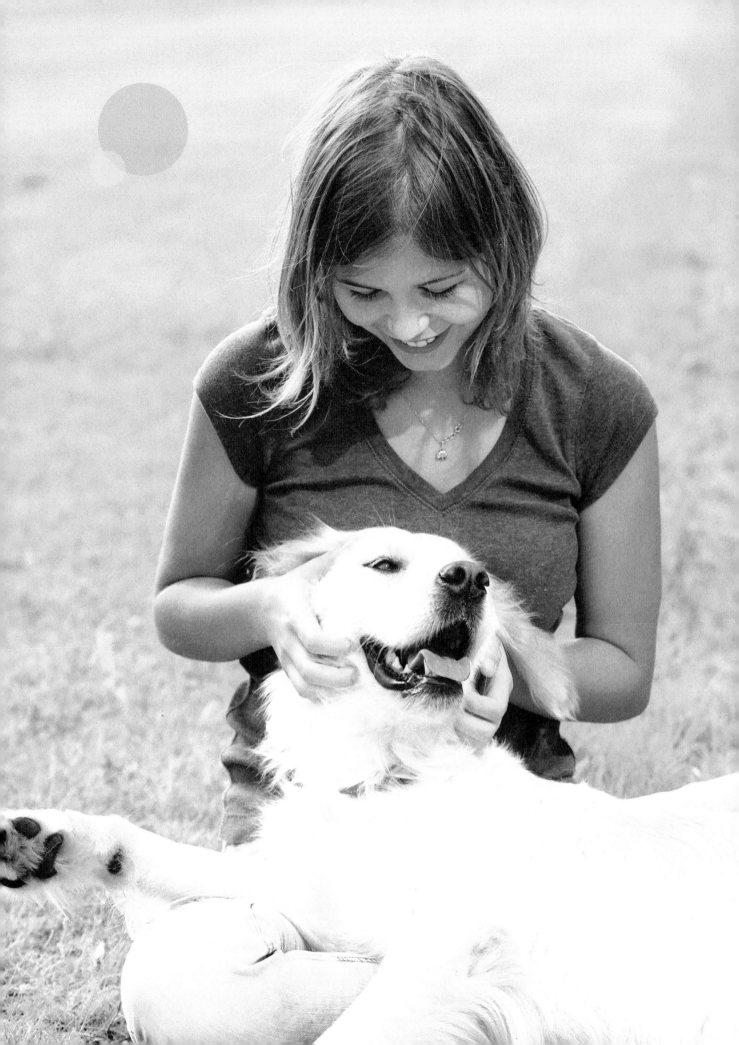

Contents

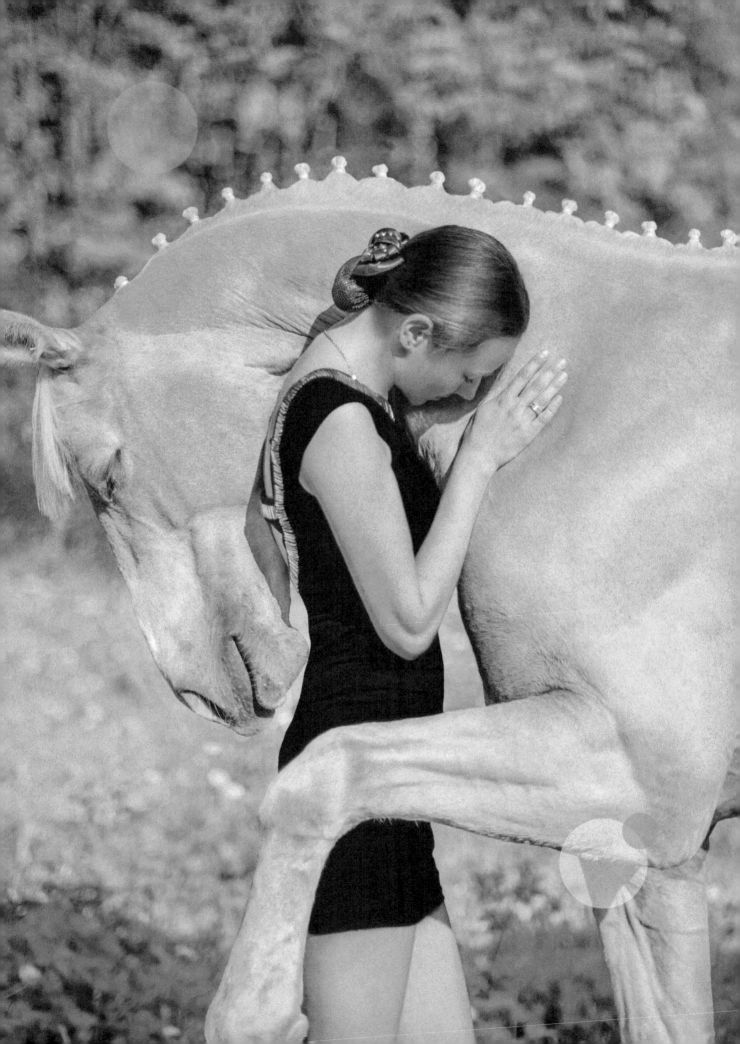

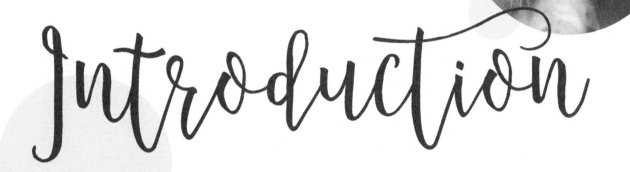

Introduction

WHAT IS THE ANIMAL METHOD OF MEDITATING WITH ANIMALS?

What if you could easily tune in to your pet's comforting, healing, and constant love and, in doing so, tap into a universal calm and a more enlightened way of being in the world? This is precisely what The Animal Method allows you to do.

The Animal Method is a way of connecting more deeply with your animals through the practice of meditating with them. When you have a more conscious relationship with each other, it brings both you and your animal companion many benefits—mentally, physically, emotionally, and spiritually. Yes, even spiritually, as Dr. Marc Bekoff and other notable biologists including Jane Goodall have written about.[1] Animals sharing similar brain structures to ours are capable of spiritual experiences because they are originated from the same deep primitive parts of the brain. This is discussed in detail in the book *The Spiritual Doorway in the Brain* by Kevin Nelson, a professor of neurology at the University of Kentucky. Our uplifted energy and mood affects the animal's spirit just as we are affected by their energy and mood.[2] This is the essential teaching behind Meditating with Animals,

Meditation is for everyone. Animals are the teachers we have directly in front of us.

and therefore also The Animal Method. It's a fun and mind-opening approach that works to change your habits from being routine everyday activities to being in-the-moment meditations with your animals. Through the use of simple and practical meditations that enhance connection, you can improve the way you relate to and support each other, opening the door to all the benefits that Meditating with Animals can provide.

While meditation can be hard for many of us and we can find ourselves wondering if we're doing it correctly and getting all the benefits, we need only look to our animals for guidance, because they are doing it all the time—they are always in the present moment. They were not taught or influenced in any way to achieve their meditative states; they are simply *being*. We humans are also creatures of this earth, and it is possible for us to achieve a similar state of presence and meditativeness that our animal companions do. And we have the ideal opportunity to learn how to do this through our relationships with our animal companions.

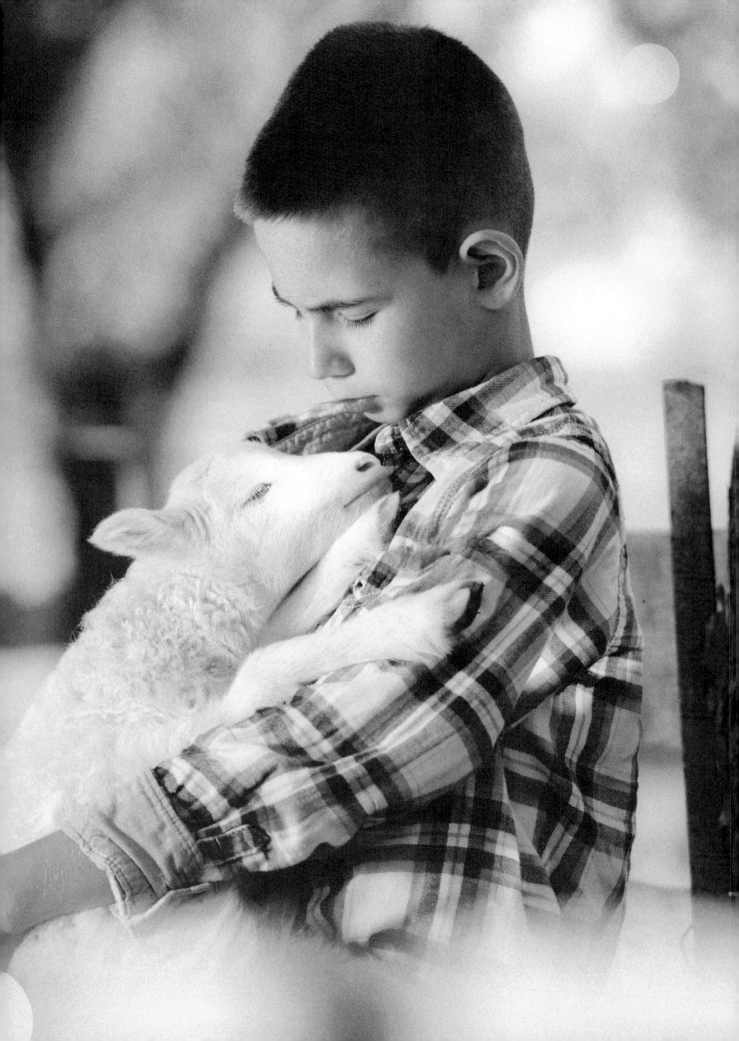

Animals are always in the present moment. They were not taught or influenced in any way to achieve their meditative states; they are simply being.

The Animal Method is something that came to me during my journey of recovery from a relentless series of personal challenges, which began with the discovery of thyroid cancer two days after I returned home from my mother's funeral. Following the surgery to remove my thyroid gland and the cancerous masses attached to it came the final breakdown of my marriage: separation and divorce. My "recovery" period was further hampered by the loss of my voice and difficulty breathing, due to a vocal cord being damaged and paralyzed during the surgery. This required another operation to repair it. I received radioactive iodine treatment and then began dealing with the complexities that came with my body adjusting to the thyroid replacement medication while simultaneously, I had to deal with the sale of my home, coordinate my third move in two years, participate in the sale of my businesses, determine how I was going to start my life over and make a living, and, even more heartbreakingly, grieve the sudden death of one of my cherished animal companions, Sophie, of fifteen years. All of this happened within a very short period of time.

No longer having the support of my mother and my husband forced me to reconnect with myself. In doing so, I unearthed my own powerful and protective instincts for healing—the strength that lay dormant inside me, ready for this awakening, and a lifetime of wisdom that was waiting to be tapped into for my accelerated growth and expansion. And the unconditional love and constant presence of my animals were instrumental during this period of my life. It was then that I also realized how animals had *always* been the refuge in my life. My home was not safe for me—I grew up with a physically, mentally, and emotionally abusive father and a mother who was a victim of this same abuse and therefore unable protect me. To survive, I tried to make myself invisible and turned to my animals for comfort and love.

The healing and energetic exchanges I experienced from them was the salve to my soul. But now as an adult, I noticed how hard they were working to heal me, I became concerned that taking their energy depleted them of theirs, and I wondered how I could return that healing energy to them in a conscious act of recycling. The Animal Method is a teaching that was gifted to me by my animals so that I could do exactly that. It's something I conceived of when I began to explore the power of meditating with my animals. I am eternally grateful to them for this, and my intention in writing this book is to share this gift of understanding with others in order to help people and animals everywhere comfort and heal each other.

BENEFITS OF THE ANIMAL METHOD

The benefits of The Animal Method are unlimited. When your mind, body, and spirit are in balance, your animal can manifest behaviors of healing, comforting, unconditional loving, and a total state of calm presence. The ultimate goal is to work in tandem so that you may benefit from the best of your animal's natural healing abilities and unconditional love while opening yourself up to joining them in that place so that they, too, can benefit from the gifts you have to offer them. And the ideal way to achieve this is through meditation. As you'll learn in the pages of this book, Meditating with Animals can take many forms, beginning with establishing a present-moment connection with them and then including sitting, walking, playing, riding, and so much

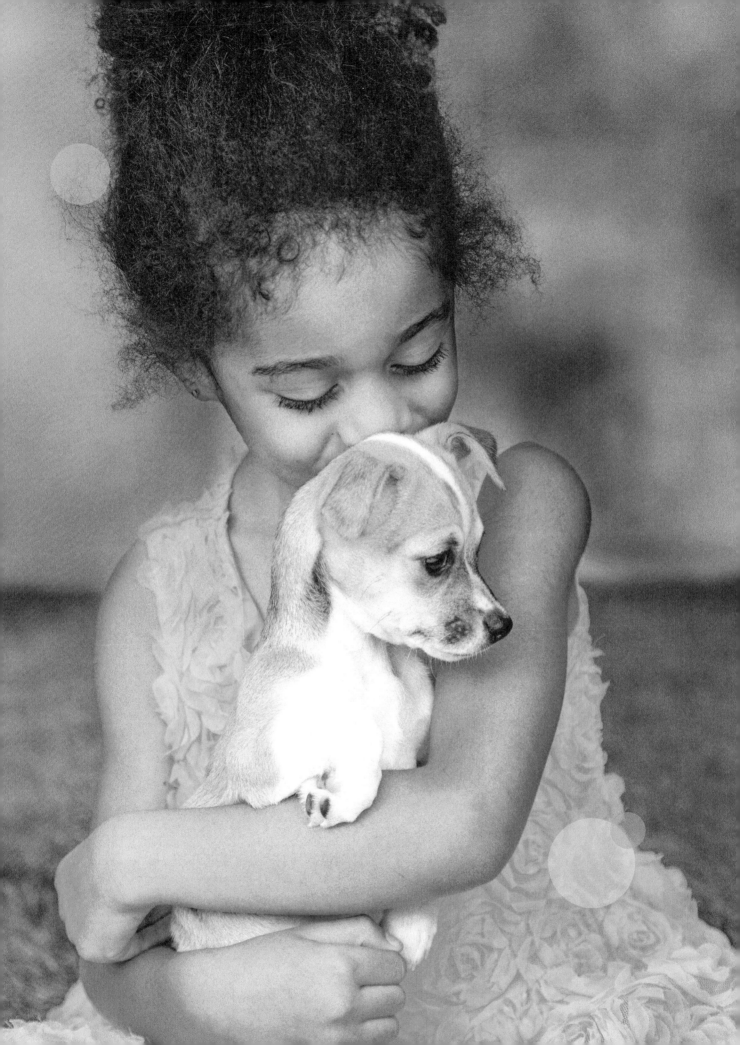

Awaken your curiosity for the possibilities of what can be, and enjoy!

more. To go deeper, you can open your heart and create a loving space to share with your animal to play, to heal, to learn, to calm, or to simply commune.

Through The Animal Method, you will discover that one of your greatest sources of healing is your relationship with your animal. Learning to meditate with them can bring relief from stress, worry, fear, anxiety, sadness, grief, illness, loneliness, relationship problems, addictions, and more. Incorporating the practice into your daily life will lead to peace of mind, a sense of well-being, and a sense of compassion and connection—to them, ourselves, our friends and family, nature . . . and, ultimately, the universe.

There is a reason why we chose our animal companions or why they chose to be with us. They are one of nature's greatest gifts to us and they hold this noble job with great responsibility without question or limitations. It can be our honor and our joy to return these gifts in kind to them, creating a reciprocal exchange of soothing grace.

HOW THIS BOOK IS ORGANIZED

Within the seven steps that make up the chapters of this book, I will share with you how to discover the reasons to be in awe of your animal (Step 1), how to notice what your animal is sensing and use your own senses likewise (Step 2), how to go more fully into the present moment with them (Step 3), how to discover and explore the possibilities for meditating with your animals (Step 4), how to see that you can nurture your animal and yourself when you allow yourself to slow down (Step 5), how to give and receive unconditional love (Step 6), and finally, how to learn to stay in stillness with your animal in order to have more meaningful connections with them (Step 7). The chapters provide meditation exercises specially designed to help you achieve each step: **A**we, **N**otice, **I**n the Moment, **M**editate, **A**llow, **L**ove, and **S**tay.

By sharing The Animal Method in this book, I hope to help you begin to see more clearly the teacher, the healer, the magical being who is right there at your feet and who is also within you! Once you have opened the door to Meditating with Animals, you will find that you can do this naturally—and your connections with your animals will never be the same. What you will learn will improve the health and well-being of both you and your animal companion.

—**PAMELA ROBINS**

Founder, Meditating with Animals™ and The Animal Method™

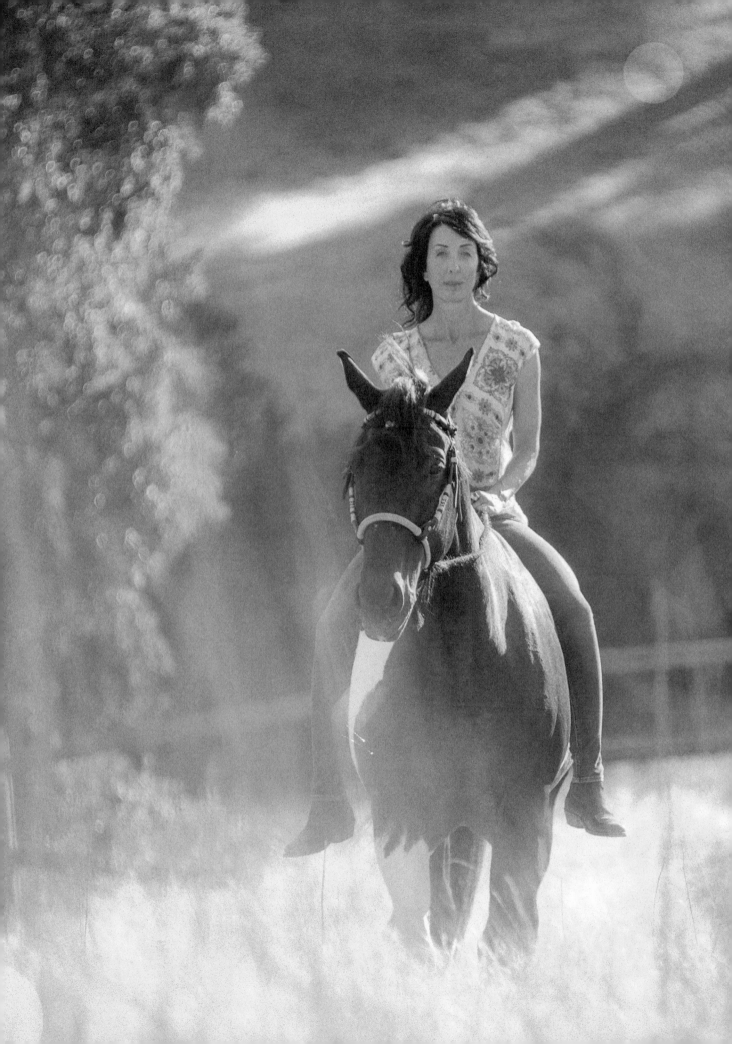

Awe **A** **N** **I**

In the
moment

Notice

Meditate Love

M A L S

Stay

Allow

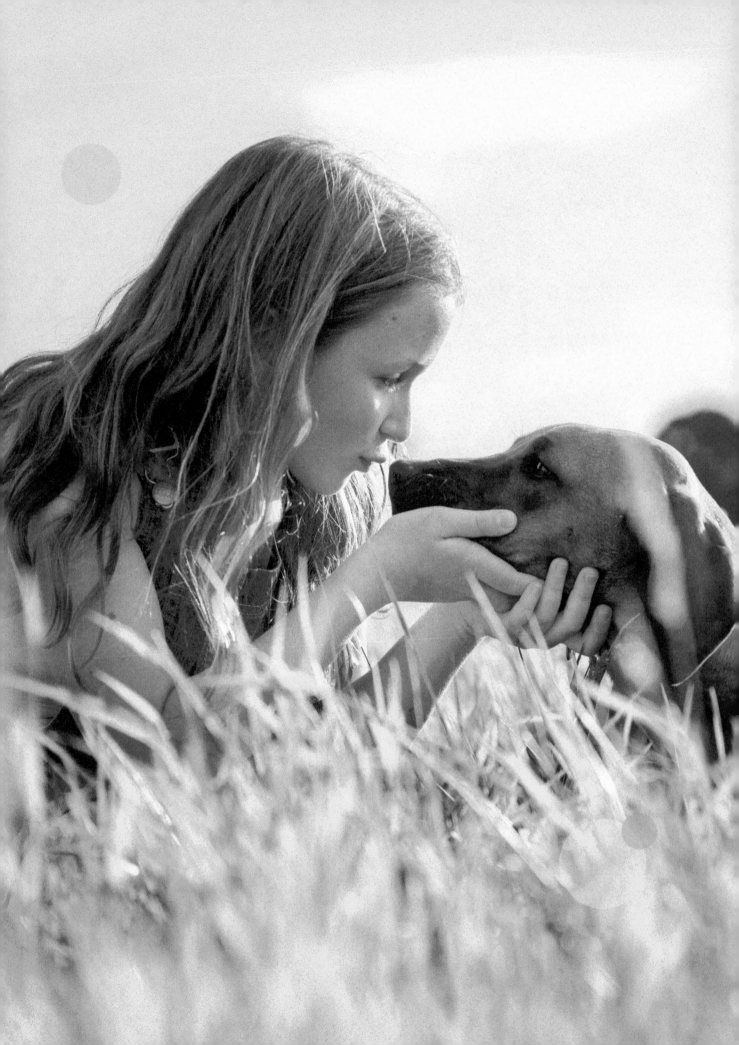

step one

Awe

finding reasons
to be in **AWE**
of your animal

the real voyage of discovery consists not in seeking new landscapes but in having new eyes.

—MARCEL PROUST

The world is full of magic things, patiently waiting for our senses to grow sharper.

—W.B. YEATS

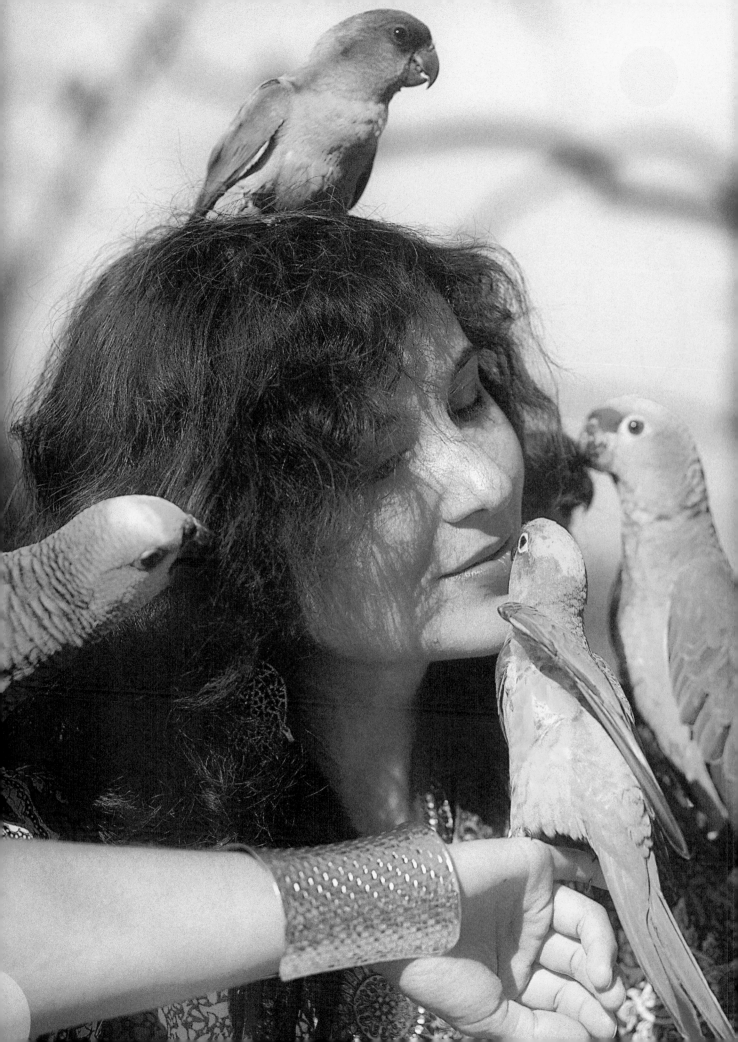

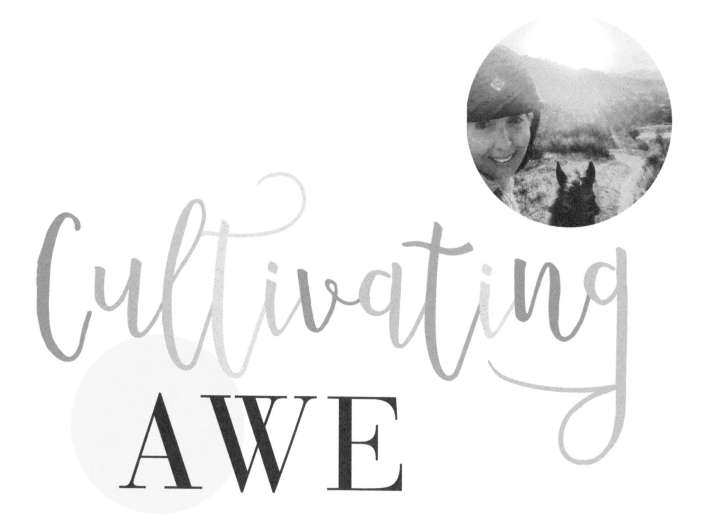

Cultivating AWE

THE FEELING OF AWE CAN GIVE US JOY, LOVE, CALMNESS, AND ELATION, and can even take our breath away—a natural high! There is science behind what the feelings of awe do to uplift us and bring increased health into our lives and relationships, which I'll get into more shortly. And I will also, of course, discuss how we benefit from the awe that our animals make us feel, but I want to begin by naming a few awesome things that we come across in the course of our day that we may have stopped noticing or we maybe even take for granted to some extent.

Isn't it awesome that we are alive and that the complex internal workings of our bodies allow us to do so many wonderful things every single day? Isn't it awesome to have family and friends whom we are able to text or call anytime we want to connect? And how awesome is it that there are vehicles that start up with a key or the push of a button and then you can drive . . . anywhere? It's awesome that buildings and homes have been designed and constructed to provide shelter and protection for us, with electricity and heat and air conditioning. Awesome that airplanes can fly us to other parts of our planet; that our planet floats in space; that the sun lights up our world and warms us; that the moon illuminates our nights and the stars hang above us in the sky. The world is full of so many awesome things: the mountains, the ocean, the clouds, and the many moods of Mother Nature, including powerful extremes such as hurricanes, tornadoes, and earthquakes.

Awe seems to be a universal emotion, but it has been largely neglected by scientists— until now.

—MELANIE RUDD

We are awesome, and we are surrounded by awesome. This can make us lose the awe we once had, so it's up to us to discover it again or seek out awesomeness from time to time so we can appreciate the phenomenal contributions that the minds of others have made in our lives as well as those that nature has given us. Just writing this very short list made me feel appreciation and gratitude for all I have, all I am able to do, and for simply existing. A wondrous yet calm feeling came over me: awe.

There's a quotation by Suzy Kassem that I love because it really defines the importance of wonder and awe: "The key to a wonderful life is to never stop wandering into wonder." It's also easy enough to remember and recall as a mantra for ourselves. So, just as we should take the time to appreciate the awesomeness in our own lives, we can and should also appreciate the awesomeness of the animals in our lives and those around us in nature.

THE SCIENCE

BEHIND THE BENEFITS

of Feeling Awe

THE SCIENCE OF AWE AND HOW IT IS RELATED TO OUR HEALTH AND well-being has been the subject of studies conducted by Dacher Keltner of the University of California, Berkeley, and Jonathan Haidt of New York University. Their emerging research suggests that there are indeed beneficial consequences of awe that may extend to our physical health, which is very exciting because awe is available to all of us through our animals.[3]

While this is good news, Keltner and Haidt also found a link between negative emotions and poor health issues such as heart disease, in addition to shorter life spans. What they are discovering through their research is that inflammation may

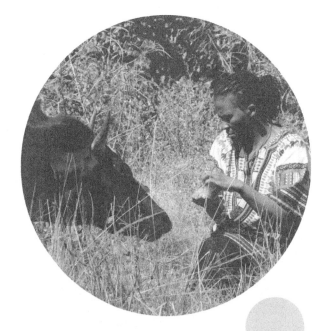

be partially responsible for this link. They believe it has to do with the molecules involved in inflammation, known as interleukin-6 (IL-6), which are essential for our body's response to infection and injury. High levels of these molecules in our bodies over a long period of time were identified in the case of many different kinds of illnesses, ranging from diabetes to depression.

Interestingly, there have not been many studies focused on the health effect of positive emotions, and so a team at the University of Toronto led by Jennifer Stellar (who was also involved in studying awe in Keltner's lab at Berkeley) set out to investigate the connection. In one particular study, they asked ninety-four students to fill out questionnaires aimed at determining how often they had experienced various emotions during the past month. The scientists assessed the various levels of that inflammation-promoting IL-6 molecule by collecting saliva samples from each student. What they found was that more positive emotion was associated with lower levels of IL-6. Stellar said of the research, "We know positive emotions are important for well-being, but our findings suggest they're also good for our body."[4]

And so it would seem that it's in all of our best interests to lead a healthier, less stressful life in which a positive emotion like awe plays a big part. And we are more likely to experience awe if we have the energy to seek it out purposefully—a stronger desire to discover new things, go places, and make new connections. Without this energy and desire, a person can retreat inward and become withdrawn or depressed. The great news is that if you have an animal companion there is already something awesome in your life, and I will now show you how to tap into that wonderful resource.

Finding the
AWE
IN ANIMALS

I LIVE IN THE MOUNTAINS NOW, AND SO I HAVE AN ABUNDANCE OF
wildlife crossing my path on a daily basis: animals such as horses, donkeys, rabbits, birds, squirrels, coyotes, and snakes. When I lived in the jungle in Mexico it was parrots, scorpions, lizards, coatimundi, and tarantulas, just to name a few! When I lived in a big city, it was mostly pigeons and rats. Wherever I am, I notice the wildlife around me and have always found awe in the way they are able to survive in our world.

Many of us need not look outside of our own homes to have an awesome animal encounter—we have our animal companions right beside us to experience this with. For example, you could look at your dog and think about the fact that history can trace the origins of canine domestication back thirty thousand years in the Upper Paleolithic of Europe. Here in the Americas, animal domestication can be traced back to about eleven thousand years ago.[5] Personally, I like to take this big step back and view my cats as being connected to their wild ancestors, understanding that this lineage runs through them and is part of who they are. Then I think about how they interact with me: eating, sleeping, playing, and communicating to me in their language. I have two rescue cats from the Yucatán jungle in Mexico, and I find it particularly awesome to be their guardian. It fills me with awe to know I am able to have such a close bond with animals that were once feral.

To help inspire your own awe of the animal companions you may have in your life, I've gathered below some awesome facts about cats and dogs and their wild instinctual behaviors.

AWESOME FACTS ABOUT CATS!

Domestic cats carry with them wild traits, especially their hunting instincts. A great example of this is cats bringing their owners dead birds or mice, which is something I've experienced firsthand. It happened many years ago when I lived in Brooklyn, New York. I was the recipient of a dead bird one morning while I was still sleeping. Right on the bed, blood and all, our cat, Tripp, made the special delivery. When I awoke and saw it, I knew it was a gift and felt honored and horrified all at once.

Why do our cats do this? It's because even though cats have been domesticated, they are not much different from their ancestors. Female cats have an instinct to teach their babies how to eat their food, which you'll see them do in the wild by bringing home injured or dead prey. If they have been spayed, female cats might not have youngsters to impart their hunting techniques to, but they still possess their natural impulses to act out their role as a mother and teacher. And this is when you, as a family member, are chosen as the recipient of this very important wisdom.[6] Which is awesome! Offering your cat a nice "thank you" in appreciation and gratitude for

It is in this simple desire to connect with their greatness that we can discover something new about their wild nature.

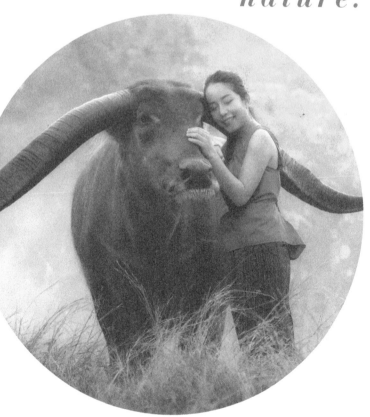

sharing this gift before removing it would be an acknowledgment of how your cat views you and wants to interact with you being in their world and not vice versa.

Ever wonder why your cat makes those fascinating chattering or twittering noises when they are sitting in the window watching birds or squirrels? Some experts think that the sound they are making is an exaggeration of the "killing bite," which is what happens when a cat captures her prey by the neck and snaps the bones by working her teeth through them.[7] Whoa. That's very awesome!

AWESOME FACTS ABOUT DOGS!

Even though the exact origin of our four-legged dog friends is still a bit of a mystery, many commonplace canine behaviors can be explained by looking at the behaviors of wolves.

Tamar Geller, a life coach for dogs and their people, has observed wild wolf packs in their natural habitats. This is her explanation of the reason why a dog will jump on you and "greet" you when you return home: "It is because in wolf packs, when a pack leader returns from hunting the young cubs jump and lick the bigger wolf's lips. That action causes the hunting wolf to regurgitate food so that the cubs can eat." Geller goes on to say that interestingly, our response to this behavior should be to turn our back so the dog knows we don't have anything, rather than reprimanding them for what comes naturally.[8] So basically your dog wants to lick your face off because he is checking to see if you have any food for him. When you understand the reason for this action, you can see how awesome it really is and in turn react differently.

You may have wondered why when a dog finds just the right spot to do his duty, it is usually followed by dramatic and fervent scratching and kicking of the ground in the immediate area with his hind feet. What he is actually doing is sending a double message: marking his territory not only by the smell of what he's leaving behind but also by making a big production of it so that it will be seen by those around him.[9] OK, you got that awesome message across!

THE FACT THAT WE LIVE WITH DOMESTICATED ANIMALS WHO HAVE wild instincts still running through their veins is quite remarkable. Taking the time to be in awe of something they do (that we might have initially felt we had already seen, knew, or understood) can actually take us outside of own heads and into theirs.

And so, become curious about the *why* that is behind their actions! Take a few minutes to look up something about your animal's behavior online. It is in this simple desire to connect with their greatness that we can discover something new about their wild nature. This can lead to the feeling of how awesome it is to not only to have a relationship with our animals but also that they live in our homes, our minds, and our hearts.

THE
Healer

WHEN SPEAKING ABOUT THE AWE-INSPIRING EFFECT OF OBSERVING animals, I can't offer a better example than my cat Sylvester.

He came into my life when I was living in Mexico in a house in the jungle. One day I heard a terrible shrieking cry and went to see what it was. Outside the door in the courtyard was a scrawny and very upset cat who was screaming. She would not stop.

"What am I supposed to do here?" I asked myself. I knew I had to do something—she was demanding attention and clearly needed help. I thought "OK, if you feed her, then she is your responsibility." Accepting this, I ran to get some food, much to the dismay of my indoor cats at the time, Sophie and Striped Cat. I quickly explained to them that they had all of their needs met and they were safe, loved, and cared for, whereas this cat was not as fortunate and so it was now our responsibility—for whatever reason—to help her. Or at least try. Most importantly, I needed to calm her down because her intensity was anxiety-invoking, to say the least. If another few minutes passed, I felt like I would be out there screaming with her. Something was definitely up.

So I fed her. She became quiet and ate in such a voracious manner I wondered when the last time this poor kitty had had any food. I put out some water and a little towel for her to lie down on. With her now quiet and no longer hungry I quietly tiptoed away ... backwards.

About ten minutes later, out of curiosity, I went to check on her; I couldn't help myself. I was completely shocked by what I saw: she had brought back five tiny kittens and was nursing them on the towel I had put out! My first thought was, *Oh my goodness, this is amazing!* Then, *What am I going to do with all of these animals?* Sheer panic.

Thankfully, my dear friend Claudia

This cat was not as fortunate and so it was now our responsibility... to help her. Or at least try.

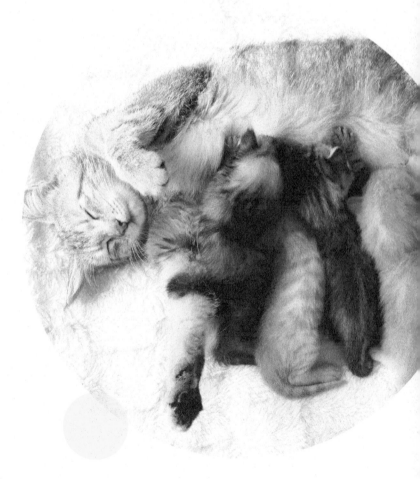

I felt this shock in my heart when the little black and white one looked into my eyes. It was in that split second that our inseparable bond began.

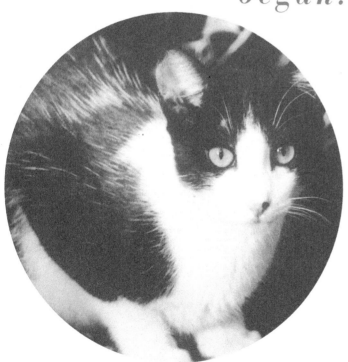

was the local vet. I participated in a trap, release, or find-a-home program with her to try to help the feral cat population in my neighborhood. When I called Claudia and told her what happened, she said the kittens were too young to bring in to have spayed and neutered and so I should wait another few weeks, feeding them in the meantime, then bring them in. So that's what I did.

A few days after their operations I picked up the kittens. On the drive home, when I turned my head around quickly to look at all of them in the backseat, I felt this shock in my heart when the little black and white one looked into my eyes. It was in that split second that our inseparable bond began. Our souls recognized each other and became forever joined. After that, I knew I could not live without him, and he became Sylvester. I ended up also taking in his sister, whom I named Beauty School, and I found homes for the others.

Throughout our (so far) thirteen years together, Sylvester has been my love, my healer, my companion, my angel, my safe place, and a selfless giver of his warm,

He reads me and acts, whatever my needs are — he just knows

comforting body, which I hold on to for dear life at times. He reads me and reacts accordingly, whatever my unspoken needs are—he just knows. When I broke my collarbone and was recovering in bed (binge-watching *Mad Men* episodes on Netflix), he climbed up and laid right on my collarbone. Mind you, Sylvester's not small and my bone was severely broken, but I was in awe that he put himself there and was doing what came instinctually to him to heal me. Despite the pain, it was kind of hard to ask him to move!

It was later that I discovered these astonishing facts: cats purr both when they inhale and when they exhale according to a consistent pattern and frequency between 25 and 150 hertz. This phenomenon has been studied with fascinating results: the particular frequency range can improve bone density and promote healing.[10] This suggests to me that Sylvester had instinctually sensed what was wrong with me and was trying to heal it! Now that is completely awesome.

When my heart has been broken, or when it just simply hurts with feelings of sadness, loneliness, or pain, Sylvester will lay his head right on my heart when he

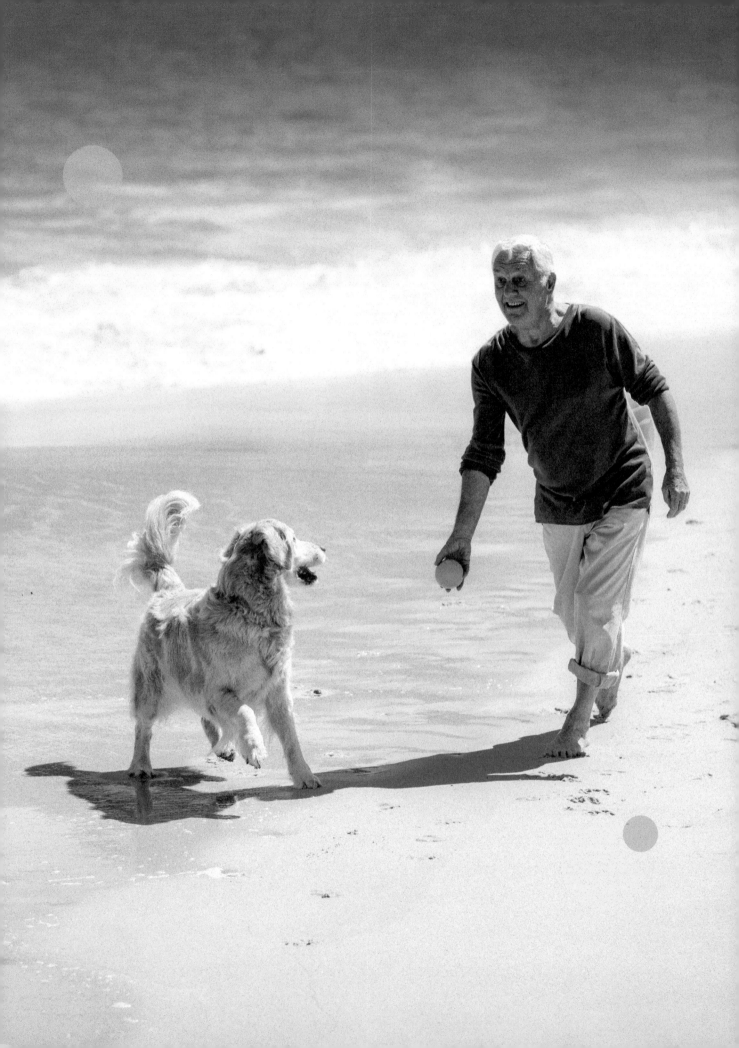

curls up beside me or on me. He very often puts his paw on my heart. I am in complete awe of his knowingness and his ability to tune into whatever emotional or physical things I'm dealing with and try to heal them. In fact, it takes my breath away.

Though I know I can't stop time, I savor every second of these interactions with mindful appreciation, looking beneath the surface to try to understand how he can have such keen awareness. Sometimes it is just so astonishing and I fill with such excitement over the profound nature of the connection that I almost ruin it by moving or wanting to exclaim out loud, "How do you know to do this, are you psychic?!"

It is exactly this moment that I switch to being gracious in order to allow Sylvester the freedom to give what he feels is needed and for me to accept it. If I can breathe and relax, I am then able to return my awe-inspired energy to him. I visualize it like millions of sparkling bubbles of excitement traveling right back into his being.

IF WE SEE—I MEAN REALLY *SEE* HOW OUR ANIMALS TRY TO NATURALLY heal us, whether it is simply how they place themselves in physical relation to us or the myriad other things they do to pull us out of ourselves and into their perspective—then we can elevate our interactions and experience the gifts we have for each other more fully.

See your animal and the things they do with awe (or aww) and feel the excitement, the softening, then the opening of the connection that develops in the space where you step outside of yourself. Pure appreciation for this free-willed spirit that you have the honor of caring for and who cares for you in your life together.

Remember, awe feels good for our spirit and our bodies respond positively from receiving it. Following is a meditation I recommend for inspiring feelings of awe between you and your animal.

THE *Awesome* MEDITATION

START BY LOOKING AT YOUR ANIMAL. CHOOSE SOMETHING THAT YOU love about him or her; something you find beautiful, unique, amazing, or incredible that fills you with awe.

Example: Right now, Sylvester is curled up sleeping next to me. I am in awe that he feels safe and finds comfort being close to me when there are many other places he could go to seek out peace or his own comfort.

- Relax and focus on your chosen reason for awe. There most likely is a feeling that rises up into your heart, and you might find yourself smiling. Hold that thought and feeling with you as you close your eyes.

- Take at least twelve deep inhales followed by twelve deep exhales.

- If your animal is within arm's reach, you can put your hand on them. The touch of your hand carries your energy and intentions.

- Send your animal thoughts of appreciation and love for who they are and why they are awesome to you.

- It's OK and completely normal that other thoughts will come into your mind. Allow them to come on in and, when they do, turn them around and send them back out, replacing them once again with a loving thought or feeling of appreciation for your animal.

- To help you maintain the connection with your animal, focus on the feel of their fur, the warmth of their body, pattern of their breathing, or a sigh, snore, or purr.

- Continue to breathe in and out, finding oneness with the body of life at your side.

- Notice that through this connection you can experience the animal's natural state of being as your own.

- Try to sit with them for twenty to thirty minutes, if not more, so they can really absorb this softened energy with you.

- Enjoy these awesome moments together!

This is a great meditation to do at night when you are falling asleep, a time when many animals like to be in bed with us. I love to drift off with my hand on one or both of my cats, feeling grateful and in awe that we are all together as a family finding comfort in each other.

It's such a peaceful way to end the day!

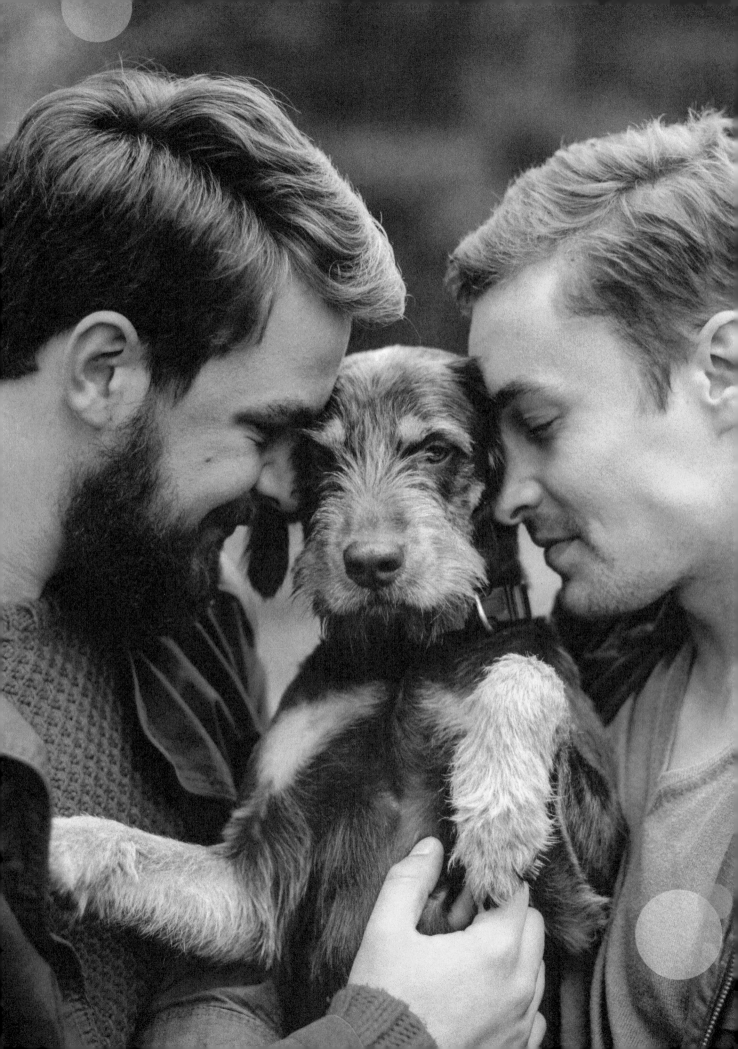

step two

NOTICE

using your senses to **NOTICE** what your animal is experiencing, and then joining them

Attention
is the rarest
and purest
form of
generosity

—SIMONE WEIL

The most precious gift we can offer anyone is our attention. When mindfulness embraces those we love, they will bloom like flowers.

—THICH NHAT HANH

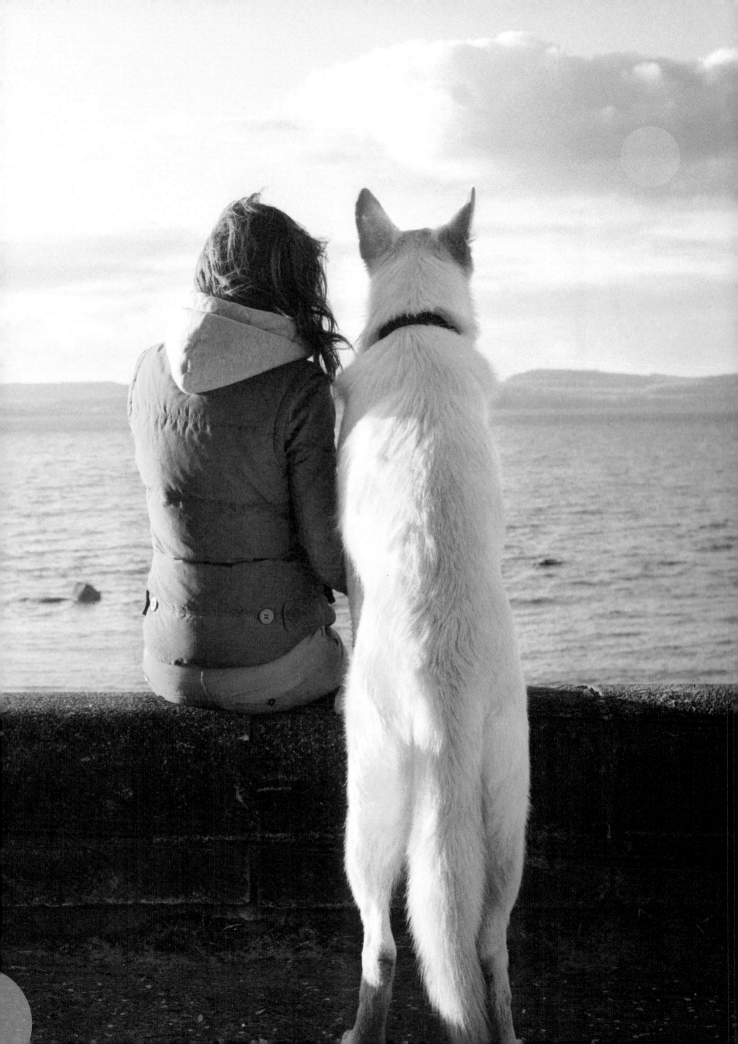

A window
INTO YOUR ANIMAL'S
SOUL

IF WE TAKE THE TIME TO STAND BACK AND WATCH THE THINGS OUR animals naturally do, it can provide us with a window into their soul. Animals have free will. They think. They feel. They are curious. They can become scared or surprised. They can be very funny—hilarious even! They can become tired or not feel well. They can get bored. They can get excited!

If you choose to *notice*, then you can find wonder in the smallest of details. For example, when I notice my cat sleeping, a quiet joy fills my heart as I see his eyes flutter, his body moving with the rise and fall of his breath, or perhaps a twitching tail or whiskers. I like to count the dots on his cheeks where his whiskers grow or the stripes that wrap around his little arms, admiring the intricate patterns and texture of his fur.

Take time to observe things like how your animals look, feel, and behave. When you do, keep in mind that our animals have unique and incredible ways of navigating their surroundings, of which we are a part. Similar to humans, animals use at least five different sensory methods of assessing their environment: sight,

If you choose to notice, then you can find wonder in the smallest of details.

sound, touch, taste, and smell.[11] Animals do not perceive the environment in the same way a human would, and different animals use their senses in different ways. Following are a few examples.

If you observe a horse, you can tell exactly what he or she is looking at and where their concentration is—even how they feel—just by watching their ears! Depending on where their attention is directed, a horse's ears will be facing forward, backward, or sideways—whichever position will allow them to best hear what they are focused on. The ears are almost always active. If both ears are forward, the horse is paying attention to something in front of them. If the ears are casually moving about, the horse may be relaxed and just checking things out or attempting to tune in to something specific and home in on it. Pinned-back ears is a sure sign a horse is angry or upset.

I like to talk or sing to my horse, Tuxedo, and when I do it makes me smile to see his ears moving around listening to me. A horse's ears are able to move a full 180 degrees because they have the use of ten different muscles that allow them to do so (in comparison, the human ear has only three muscles), and they can single out a targeted area to tune in and listen to. Hearing is so important for a horse's

When you notice their opinion, mood, and communication, you can choose to go with it and smile at whatever it may be.

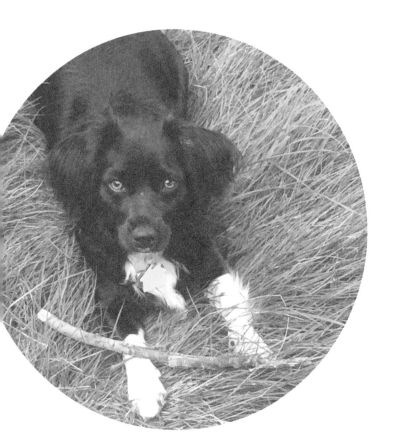

survival. When they position the ears in the direction of a noise, they are better able to determine if it is a threat or not.[12] By using this incredible feature, Tuxedo can detect something off in the distance well before I become aware of it or even see it. Knowing this keeps me on my toes and very aware of my surroundings when I am riding him.

If it's your cat that you are observing, be mindful that their eyesight is truly extraordinary, especially their peripheral vision. A cat's pupils can dilate wider to capture a panoramic view of the landscape. They are also specialists in sensing the tiniest of movements, a hunting skill developed over thousands of years. Where cat vision is particularly intense is at nighttime. Compared with humans, cats have six to eight times more rod cells in their eyes, enabling them to detect light at very low levels, so they can see things in the dark that we cannot.[13]

When it comes to dogs, their sense of smell is very different than is ours. In fact, the part of a dog's brain that is devoted to analyzing smells is forty times larger than that of a human! Incredibly, their sense of smell is about ten thousand times more acute than ours.[14]

The idea is to look at your animal companion and notice *how they notice* the world around them and how they react to it. This includes their reactions to you.

As anyone who's ever had a dog knows, when you are getting ready to take your dog for a walk, he or she will sense your energy and intention, and they will react accordingly. Most dogs love going out for walks and so they will get very excited, while some don't like walks at all or may just not be in the mood at that moment, in which case they will object to the idea by sitting down and refusing to move, possibly running away from you or even hiding!

When I was a child I had a dachshund named Heidi, whom I desperately wanted to walk around the neighborhood. She'd seem alright with this idea until we got right down to the end of the driveway, and then she would sit. Nothing I did could get her to walk with me from that point on. Ever. In this way, Heidi made it clear to me that her idea of a walk was a slow and reluctant excursion down to the end of the driveway followed by a fast-as-you-can-move-your-legs run back to the house. A total of four minutes! I never forced her, I'd just bring her back inside and let her do what she preferred, which was to have tea and cookies with my mother, on her lap . . . watching soap operas.

When you pay attention to the opinion, mood, and communication your animal demonstrates, you are honoring the fact that your animal is a being separate from you who has his or her own needs at any given moment. If they don't show excitement for an idea you have, you can alter your plan to accommodate them just as you would a friend or partner when they don't have the same interest in something that you do.

If you sense excitement in your animal, then the answer to whatever it is you're suggesting is yes! If you sense hesitation, then the answer is probably no, and that's

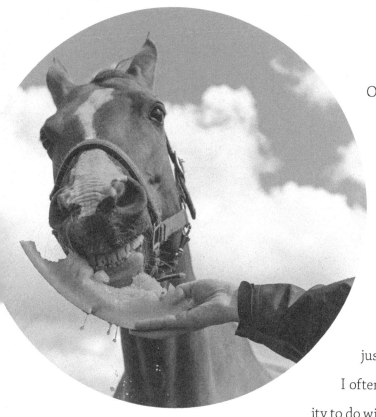

OK. Let go of your expectations and become flexible by making another choice to try something different that your animal might prefer to do. For example, if it's your dog, go through the list: Playing catch in the yard? A ride in the car to the dog park? Tea with Mom? Or try something new—get creative, just don't get stuck!

After six years of having my horse, Tuxedo, it always amazes me that when I slow down and just hang out with him like I would a human friend, I often find some new little interaction, game, or activity to do with him, or I discover something new that he likes.

I was surprised to find out that he enjoys, well . . . *loves* eating watermelon! He expressed interest when I was eating it near him one day, so I held out a piece to him to try. He showed his excitement and joy by slopping and slurping and making the biggest mess and nudging my hand for more before he finished the first half of the slice. His discovery became my entertainment, and we shared in this delight together.

Being able to notice an opportunity, to tune in, and to adapt to a changing set of circumstances is a useful practice for us not only in relation to our animal companions but to our human companions too! It can lead to fun, interesting, exciting, and new adventures . . . and in the process, we expand upon our compassionate and loving nature.

Walking
AND WAKING

I HAVE TO SAY, I NEVER THOUGHT THAT I WOULD FIND MYSELF WALK-ing a cat. My certainty of this came from observing the many cats I'd lived with throughout my life. Most of them, once indoors, very quickly got used to the luxuries: being waited upon, access to food on demand, sunlit rooms to relax in by day, a warm body to sleep beside at night, favorite hiding places, toys, treats, and usually a buddy to play around with. My cats didn't have much interest in seeing what was beyond the door when I closed it behind me to leave—with one exception.

My Kit-Ten came from the jungle in Mexico. Lake Bacalar in the southern area of the Yucatán Peninsula, to be exact. You might be wondering how we found each other! I lived in Mexico a few hours north of that area in Playa del Carmen with my (then) husband for several years. During that time, we generously supported a local cat rescue program called Coco's Animal Welfare, the founder of which, Laura, is a wonderful human being, a force of nature, and a friend. Kit-Ten was delivered to Laura's shelter one day after a kind soul had found him and his young brothers and sisters in the jungle near the lake. Some of the kittens were sick and did not make it, but Kit-Ten survived the harsh tropical conditions in the early few weeks of his life long enough to be plucked from danger, put in a carrier, and driven the three hours up the coast to the animal rescue.

At the time this happened, I was living in California (where I'd moved from Mexico a few years prior) and was suffering from the recent and very significant loss of one of my most cherished animal companions, Striped Cat, whom we'd brought back to the States with us. We had rescued him when we first moved to Mexico (more on that story later), and so I felt that rescuing another striped jungle cat from Mexico in his memory would be the perfect way to honor him.

I kept tabs on the growth of Coco's Animal Welfare by following it on Facebook. Staff members would frequently post photos of cats available for adoption, and one day I saw this little guy and just knew he was going to be with me. Luckily he was available and a volunteer was able to bring him to me on a flight to California a few weeks later.

Kit-Ten had been so well socialized during his time at the rescue, thanks to the caring staff and the fact that there'd been lots of other cats to live freely with and kind people who showed up to do "kitten cuddling" on a weekly basis. I discovered quickly that he is an incredibly confident, loving, funny, curious, fearless, and energetic little guy—with a wild streak and exotic looks to go along with his heritage. He wasted no time at all bonding with Sylvester and Sophie (my other kitties at the time) and me. I remember working on the computer at my desk the first night he was with us, and he was laying on my arm with his paws on my hand while I typed away. The next morning he curled himself up on my chest, under my chin, as I cradled him in my arm while I was having my coffee. I was in love! While Sophie "tolerated" him, Sylvester fell under his spell right away like I had. Within minutes of Kit-Ten's arrival, the two were like old friends. Since that day, Kit-Ten adores his Sylvester and they spend a lot of time curled up with each other or kitty boxing and chasing each around the house. He keeps Sylvester feeling young and healthy by making him exercise every day. It's the perfect relationship!

After Kit-Ten had been with us for a little while, I was talking one day with a friend and she mentioned a pet psychic who she felt was exceptional. I was intrigued enough to make an appointment to speak with this person about my animals. During the conversation, the psychic shared with me that Kit-Ten told her he would like to be able to go outside. As soon as I heard this, I recognized that I already knew he wanted this. I had been wishing I could let him out because he was always nearby the screened door when

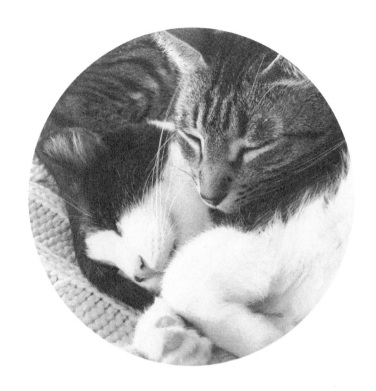

I discovered quickly that he is an incredibly confident, loving, funny, curious, fearless, and energetic little guy—with a wild streak and exotic looks to go along with his heritage.

The psychic shared with me that Kit-Ten told her he would like to be able to go outside. As soon as I heard this, I recognized that I already knew he wanted this.

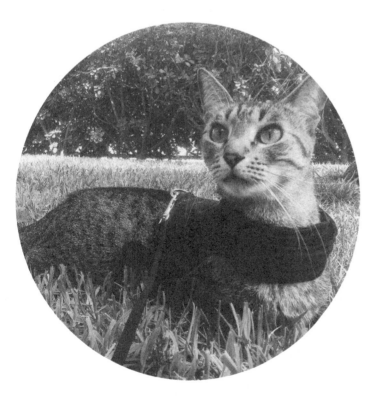

it's opened, or sometimes I would find him fixated at a window, clearly connected with and fascinated by the world outside. I just didn't know how to have him go outdoors and keep him safe, so I had put the thought aside. I lived in the mountains where there are coyotes, and so if he escaped from me he wouldn't survive under those conditions. Hearing the psychic's insight, though, it moved me to revisit the idea and figure out a way to make it a reality. I ended up finding Kit-Ten a little cat jacket that would help him realize his dream.

We tried out his jacket in the house first, and it took a few days for Kit-Ten to feel comfortable with it on. He thought it had the ability to paralyze him, and though he let me put it on him easily enough, once it was on his body he wouldn't move! When he finally attempted walking some time later, he looked like a drunken sailor—a few off-balance steps and then he'd fall down. Oh, the drama! I started to think it might not be such a good idea after all, but I continued talking with Kit-Ten and visualizing in my mind all the places we could go and the things we could do and see together when he had his "magic" jacket on. Eventually it started to change for him.

The first time I took him outside, I was a little fearful he would be able to get away from me. But I didn't want to pass that energy on to him because we were supposed to be having fun. I had made sure his jacket was secure, so I needed to settle down and relax, and I did just that by taking a few deep breaths. The fact that we were outside was really success enough for me. Kit-Ten didn't try to run away or even walk around like a dog; he allowed me to carry him out to a spot on the grass, where he laid down and smelled every micro inch of the air, dirt, and blades of grass around us. His sense of smell is very important to him and he *loves* to deeply investigate things through this sensory ability.

His attention would get pulled away from his smelling exploration by the sound of pretty much anything—a bird chirping above us in the tree or landing nearby, a squirrel, even a person walking by—and he'd focus his laser-like vision on whatever had drawn his attention. The best part was if he was surprised by something, he would puff up his tail really big, which had me laughing out loud. Very quickly, I noticed how much Kit-Ten was enjoying himself outdoors. He wasn't *overly* excited; he was just fascinated by it all and taking it all in. I started paying attention to the things he was noticing and interested in. I became

I started paying attention to the things he was noticing... I imagined him in the jungle, only a few weeks old, roaming around doing these same behaviors.

By listening through noticing, we can learn... then we can work to help bring out the best in them and allow their souls to shine and soar.

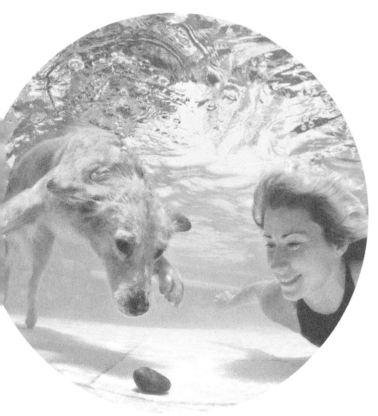

immersed in his perspective, smiling joyfully at how curious and alert he was and what he was aware of. I imagined him in the jungle, only a few weeks old, roaming around doing these same behaviors.

The next few times we ventured outside, Kit-Ten became more comfortable and bold. I discovered that he loves when people come up to him to admire and pet him. As I walked with him (which still today is kind of like a long, slow, slinky, panther-hunting-prey kind of walking), I naturally shifted into seeing the world from his perspective. He was not on my walk; I was on *his* walk.

The saying "Actions speak louder than words" holds very true when it comes to animals. By listening through noticing, we can learn what an animal is thinking about, even what they desire to do, then we can work to help bring out the best in them and allow their souls to shine and soar. My noticing created a positive change in Kit-Ten's life. It opened up a whole new world for him. Being able to facilitate this was truly an honor to be a part of and a wonderful learning experience for both of us.

He was not on my walk;
I was on
his walk.

I learned something very important from my experience with the pet psychic too. It brought out something that I had already noticed but did not act upon. Her communicating this to me put me into action. Now I know when I observe something, I have the ability to take that a step further and put it into action. In this case, the experience it led to has opened the door for me to consider taking Kit-Ten out on bigger excursions—not just outside our door. I would love for him to go to the barn to meet Tuxedo!

The connecting of the dots is very valuable for us to understand—to see how deeply we are already communicating with our animal companions and that we only need to become *just a little more* aware in order to get the whole picture, not just part of the picture.

The following meditation exercise will help you to engage in the practice of noticing what your animal is detecting and communicating with their senses, and guide you in joining them in their experience.

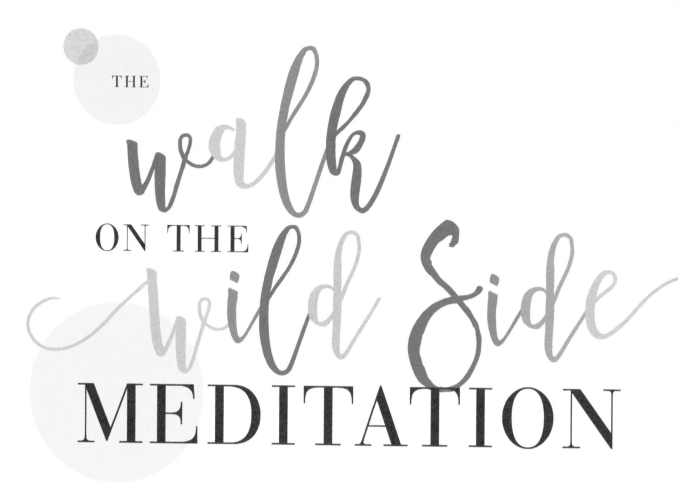

THE walk ON THE wild Side MEDITATION

THIS IS A MEDITATION YOU CAN DO WITH YOUR ANIMAL ANYTIME, BUT if you have an animal you take on walks, it's an ideal meditation to do before and during your walk. It's always a good idea to check in with yourself first to be conscious of your own energy before connecting with your animal companions. They *feel* you, and so your energy becomes their energy.

- Take a few deep breaths, breathing in love and breathing out each stress of the day, one at a time.

- It's good practice to put a name or a face, or even a situation, on those big exhales. Doing so makes it a little more effective to send those thoughts off on a ride for a little while—away from you.

- As you come in contact with your animal companion, begin to notice.

- Be aware of what you see and feel from them, just as they are doing with you.

- If the energy is positive, contagious . . . enjoy it! Notice the reaction it creates in you (perhaps it's laughter or a smile) and let that fill up your heart, then visualize returning that positive feeling to their heart.

- If your animal is worried or unsettled about something, settle your own energy even more by breathing deeply. If you are calm, confident, and stable, they will sense this. It's important not to focus on the upset from them; rather, focus on the desired outcome—calmness—and project that from yourself to your animal. When you don't feed into, take on, or allow yourself to become worried or fearful too, they will see by your actions that all is OK.

- Continue to notice your animal's energy and pay attention to what they are paying attention to, looking at it from their perspective.

- Begin to think that you are walking *as* your animal; get fully into their experience by *being* them. That's right: be your animal!

- Notice what they see, smell, hear, and react to, and what they find fun, surprising, interesting, exciting, or worrisome.

As you continue noticing you will become fully available to them, in their experience, adjusting your energy and reactions to their experiences and needs accordingly. That is really the best gift you can give your animal: your total attention. Through that attention and noticing, you will become synchronized in your shared experience— more balanced. As you support your animal companions, they, in turn, are better able to support you.

Enjoy the journey of noticing. It's fun!

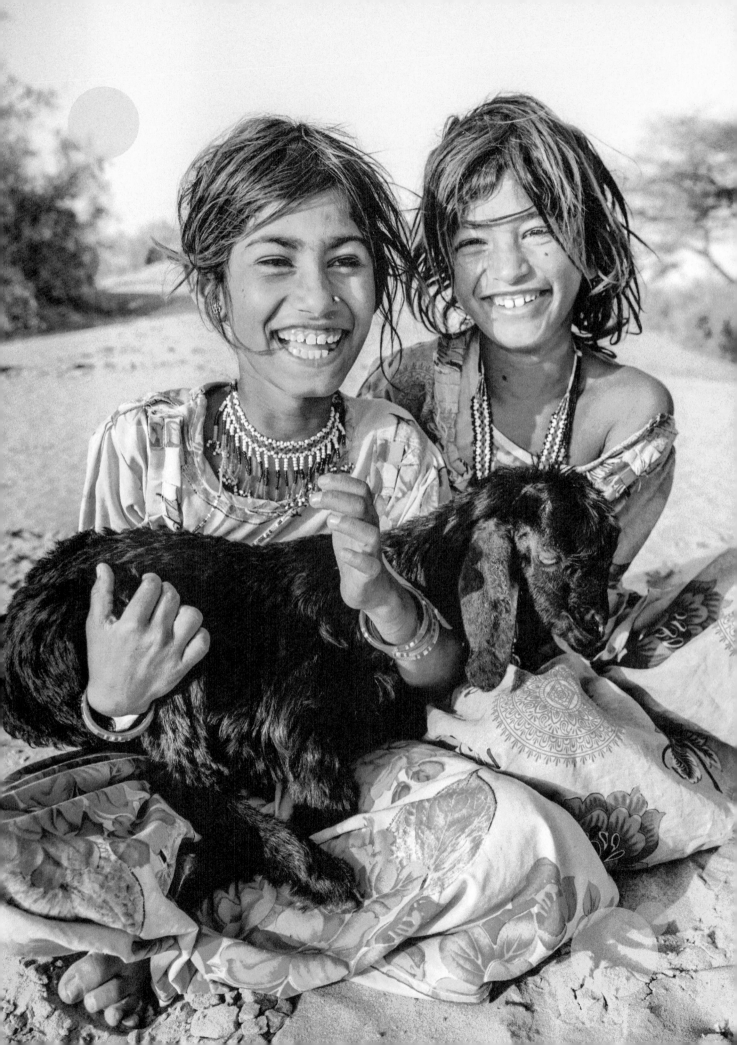

In the moment

being fully present
IN THE MOMENT
with your animal

Realize deeply that the present moment is all you ever have.

—ECKHART TOLLE

In practicing meditation, we're not trying to live up to some kind of ideal—quite the opposite. We are being with our experience, whatever it is.

—PEMA CHÖDRÖN

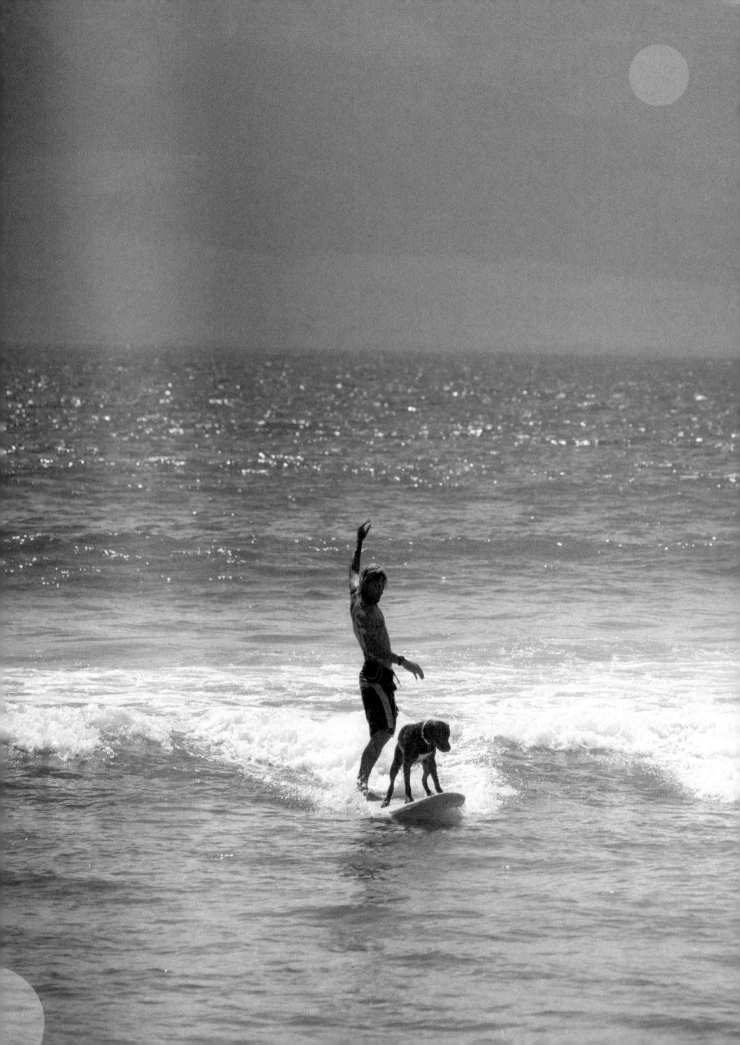

the Healers and teachers AMONG US

OUR LIVES ARE SO FULL. EVERY DAY WE ARE FACED WITH COUNTLESS issues, pressures, stresses, and deadlines. It can be overwhelming and exhausting. Many of us have suffered with health, emotional, and physical issues that arise from just trying to get through our constantly changing lives. Most of us are managing our work, families, friends, homes, and our animal companions. Because of this, it is easy to overlook the powerful antidote we have for stress right at our feet when we walk in the door at the end of another long and busy day.

The University of Missouri's Research Center for Human-Animal Interaction (ReCHAI) is exploring the many ways animals benefit people of all ages. As ReCHAI said in a statement: "Lowers blood pressure, encourages exercise, improves psychological health—these may sound like the effects of a miracle drug, but they are actually among the benefits of owning a four-legged, furry pet."[15]

While we love and are connected with our animals, we can become overwhelmed in keeping up with the tasks at hand much less adding another "activity" for our animals to our schedule. So, how do we show our love? By caring and providing for them the best way we can.

According to an *NBC News* report in 2015, the American Pet Products Association estimated that Americans would spend roughly $60 billion that year on their pets, claiming that this was mainly due to the fact that our animals are being considered family members and so the luxuries of our modern lifestyles and standards of care are being extended to them.[16] There's no question, new ways to pamper our companions are popping up every day, but I still believe the best things in life are free, such as the gift of our time and of ourselves: the deeper connection, the give and take of love and awareness, and seizing opportunities to grasp the magic that shows up in the present moment.

One of the most amazing things about our animals is that they exist in our lives without

the best things in life are free, such as the gift of our time and ourselves

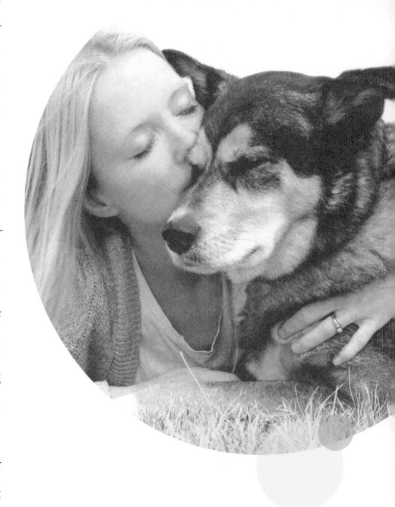

Do not dwell in the past, do not dream of the future, concentrate the mind on the present moment.

—THE BUDDHA

demanding us to do more for them than what they basically require. They are there for us when we need them and *we choose* how much time, energy, and resources to devote to them.

There's a quotation, attributed to the Buddha, which embodies the idea of how our animals can help us be more in the moment: "Do not dwell in the past, do not dream of the future, concentrate the mind on the present moment." While this isn't always easy to achieve in our hectic lives, having presence of body, mind, and spirit can provide uplifting, memorable moments for both ourselves and our animals if we just slow down long enough to see them waiting to connect with our love.

Let's go a step further. Our animal companions have subtle and not-so-subtle ways in which they communicate and express their desire to connect with us. Just as we would not ignore a person who was speaking to us, we should not ignore an animal. Just as you would try to be a good listener to a friend of yours, you can be a good listener to your animal. Yes, a dog constantly barking or a cat constantly yowling can be annoying, but they are communicating something, the same as when a baby cries.

There have been many times in my life when tuning in to the way that an animal is communicating with me has brought me more fully into the present moment. I'll share some with you now.

When Sophie, my dearly departed gorgeous green-eyed calico cat, was fifteen years old, she was so elegant and temperamental—like an aging movie star. She'd

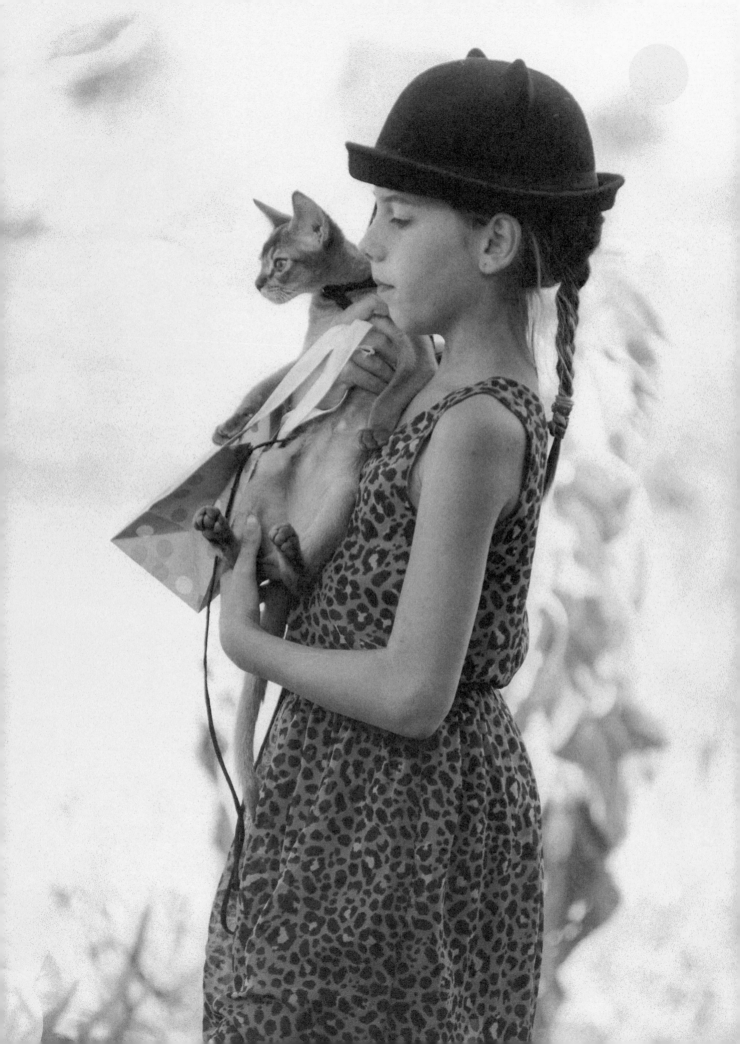

Tuxedo has changed my behavior with the phone so much that I often don't have it with me at all when I am with him.

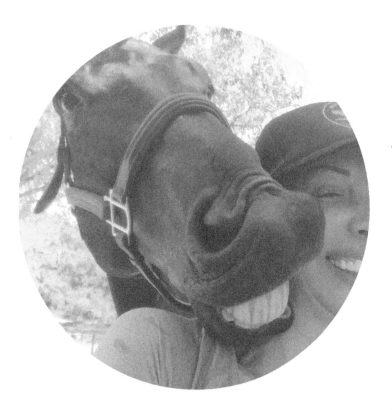

walk around the house meowing like she was practicing lines for her next feature film. She was drama itself! If one of the boys (Sylvester or Kit-Ten) even dared to look at her from across the room, she would let out a loud MEOW! And anytime she would start meowing, she wouldn't stop. None of my cajoling, pleading, or frustrated yelling "Please stop!" would change her. She had always been a talker; she just became more vocal as she aged. I was always busy trying to figure out what it was that she was talking about! Such as, meowing in front of a particular drawer in the kitchen meant "Get the brush out and brush me!" Following me around and meowing meant "I'd like a few nibbles of dry food now!" General meowing for no apparent reason meant that she either wanted my company, she didn't want the company of Sylvester and Kit-Ten (a movie star deserves her privacy after all!), she was happy to see me, or very specifically, "Please sit down, I want to be next to you." Through her constant communicating I learned a lot of different cues, and I was better able to address her many needs.

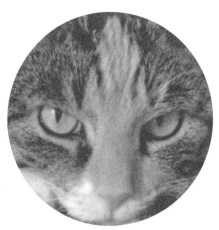

Did it lessen her talking to me? No. I think she also liked to hear herself speak. And boss us all around! She seemed to love her own voice, and now I think she was trying to tell me to find mine—which I finally have. A great lesson in patience, understanding, and communication there!

I have a little dog friend named Spangle who has quite a large dog family that surrounds her, and so when I come over she is persistent about letting me know she would like my special attention and that the other dogs need to go back to whatever they were doing before I got there. They usually do because Spangle has a lot of energy and knows what she wants—and also knows how to get it! She doesn't bark at me, but she does nudge me and stand up on her hind legs with her front paws on me, looking into my eyes with her irresistible sweet brown eyes. It's clear she wants to be picked up and held. So that is exactly what I do, and we have our love fest: she licks my face and I pet her and hold her tightly and she settles down in my arms. She has a special way of hugging, which is to really lay her body against my chest and it is such a loving and comforting gesture. Very clear communication!

Tuxedo absolutely hates it when I have my cell phone in my hand. He understands that it means he is not getting my full attention, and so he will push me with his nose, stomp his hoof, or even nip at me. He has changed my behavior with the phone around him so much that I often put it in my pocket or don't have it with me at all when I am with him. I truly feel like I am "not allowed" to use it around him. Most of my selfies (with him) are hilarious because it is his express intent to make sure I don't have an easy time getting the shot. That is crystal-clear communication!

Just being in the company of our animal companions can bring us into the present moment. It's up to us to seize these precious moments in time with them.

A Calming GESTURE

I AM, BY NATURE, A FREE SPIRIT. I HONESTLY DON'T TAKE ON ANY COM- mitments unless I'm certain that I will be able to follow through. It is one of the primary reasons I chose not to have children. I honor that part of myself that knows the level of commitment required would have been contrary to my life's path even though my heart is capable of deep, big, nurturing love.

Cats, on the other hand, I have always found to be manageable. I relate to their way of being: they are independent, they know the value of quiet companionship, and they don't require a lot of time-sensitive scheduling. And the fact that they can use a litter box rather than needing to be taken out for a walk, as dogs do, keeps it simple for me. I enjoy their comforting company, crazy antics, soft fur, wet noses, and whiskers. And I take great joy and pride in the fact that I have managed to keep those who have been in my care healthy and alive for very long periods of time!

Although I think about having a dog every single day of my existence, I have enough self-control and foresight to know that committing to that relationship would deprive me of a piece of my freedom, and I always come back to filling that space with the dogs that belong to my friends and family.

When I moved to a neighborhood that boasted a lively horse community, I was ecstatic about being around horses and having the opportunity to take riding lessons—something I had wished for since I was a little girl, following a brief period of riding at a small local farm during one summer break from school. I fell in love with Red, a darling pony whom I would endlessly take on our "adventures" around the corn field path carved out just for that purpose. I loved him so much that, much to the dismay of my family members, I refused to shower for days after returning from a visit to the barn because I didn't want to wash off his scent!

Finally, all these years later, I was able to start riding again and, in doing so, I discovered the sport of eventing, finding a passion and competitive streak that I hadn't known was inside of me just waiting to be awakened. The thought of owning a horse had never crossed my mind, so oh what a day that was when I simply got "the feeling" in my soul that I *had* to have a horse. I thought I was crazy! Talk about commitment . . . I researched, first and foremost, of course, how long horses live. I was terrified to find out that it can be up to thirty-plus years! I projected into the future what this would mean for me. Conclusion: too big of a commitment!

Despite my apprehensions about their long life spans (and much questioning of my own sanity!), the desire deep inside my soul persisted, manifesting itself in voices, images, and ideas in my head, ultimately overtaking all of my common sense. And so it was that I found myself getting a magnificent creature named Tuxedo. I had been searching daily on dreamhorse.com and then one day, there he was . . . and the words "That's my horse" came clearly into my mind.

Tuxedo is a very flashy black-and-white American Paint Horse standing at 16.2 hands who is half Thoroughbred and half Quarter Horse. He is very handsome (and he knows it!) as well as absolutely hysterical, smart, kind, grounded in who he is, brave, and talented. He loves, teaches, and heals me every day of our lives together—as I do for him. He also touches the lives of many other people and a select few animals with his gentle and charming ways. He is a magnet for meaningful, sweet interactions and I am gracious with him in recognizing and allowing him to express this part of himself beyond just with me. I jokingly say that I am in an "open relationship" with my horse. It is my honor to share his being with others without feeling the need to keep him all to myself. Our union was written in the stars long before I became aware he existed.

Committed? Yes, I'm committed—fully, madly, deeply. My love is so great at times that it feels like my heart could burst. It comes with enormous responsibility, but I just make it work, and in doing so I have discovered layers of myself that I wasn't aware lived inside me. Those discoveries never end. That is the beauty of relationships . . . continuous inquiry of oneself and another. The curiosity of it all keeps me engaged, making me feel alive and allied with myself and the universe. Having Tuxedo in my life provides me with daily gratitude for our connection. To be a leader/partner/friend with a horse astonishes me. His size, his power, his willingness to develop a deep and trusting relationship and allow me on his back is really a miracle. There are times when I have wrapped my arms around his neck and buried my face in his body, getting lost in the unbreakable bond our hearts have grown into together over the years.

Sounds a bit like a romance novel, doesn't it? But in ways it is. I never stop falling in love with him. And the love I feel for him helps me to love myself because our interactions can make me feel strong, capable, loving, and responsible yet wild, free, untamed, and adventurous. Simply put, Tuxedo makes my life more extraordinary. I've even been inspired to create an apparel line, called Horseworship, in homage to my love and admiration for him. I use large, striking fine-art photographs of horses printed on soft, stylish T-shirts and incorporate my poetry and writings on them. Tuxedo is also an inspiration to others, as evidenced by his popularity on all of my social media pages. From my own personal Facebook page to my Horseworship page on Facebook and my Meditating with Animals page on Instagram, he is everywhere! My videos and stories of our life and times together seem to speak to people; they send me e-mails letting me know how our stories have touched their lives. He is one in a million.

Like a lot of other people, I work and have a full life, yet I make time most days of the week to be with Tuxedo. Some days it's easy, but other days I don't have as much time as I would like to spend with him and I feel pressure and stress to make sure that he

The love I feel for him helps me to love myself because our interactions can make me feel strong, capable, and loving, yet wild, free, and adventurous.

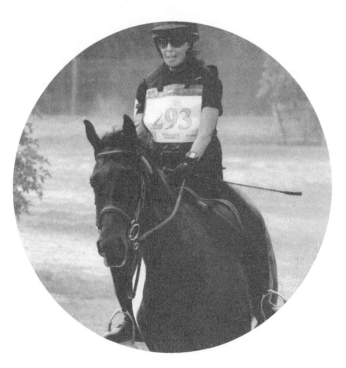

I just stopped everything and stood completely still. I started to breathe more slowly. I closed my eyes and I thanked him...

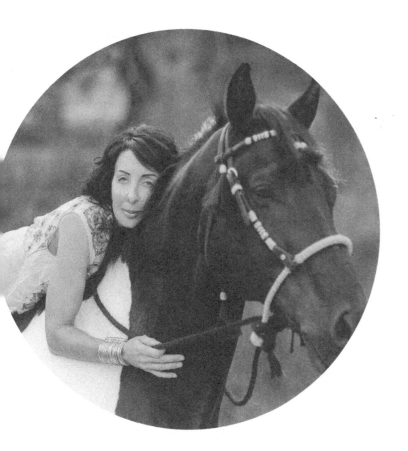

is taken care of and gets what he needs. He is a very athletic and energetic 1,200-pound animal who requires consistent exercise with varying activities (he can get bored just like we can), and his schedule includes a mix of training, playtime, and relaxation. He depends on me to make sure he gets all of these things, which is made clear by his nickering and running to greet me when I arrive. (This alone makes a trip to see him worthwhile!) Horses have energy that they must release, so just as you would take a dog to the park to run around and tire him out, you must give a horse regular opportunities to do the same. They are very much creatures of habit and thrive on routine just as our cats, dogs, birds, and other animals do. It can create a weight when you "don't have" or "can't make" the time to get your animal everything you feel they need.

I felt that way one day recently. I went to the barn thinking, "I have so many things to do and I only have an hour I can spend here." I talked to Tuxedo as I always do while grooming him, but I was rushing. He sensed this. When I went to put his bridle on, he

I was fully present in the moment.

rested his chin on my shoulder and started to breathe in my ear. I just stopped everything and stood completely still. I started to breathe more slowly. I closed my eyes and I thanked him and repeated "I love you, I love you, I love you" over and over again, melting into him. I was so grateful for his peaceful, loving gesture. I closed my eyes, and a tear drop or two fell. My heart rate lowered and I settled myself down, letting some of my stress go. I was with him. I was fully present in the moment. He offered me peaceful calmness and I returned that energy to him. I noticed what he was doing and I let it in so we could both benefit from my relaxation. I could have stood there with him forever. It made my time with him more enjoyable for both of us.

The calming gesture of Tuxedo putting his chin on my shoulder brought me into the present moment and it changed my whole day. Our animals can sense when we need to slow down and it's so important—for their sake and ours—that we take notice of the queues they give us to get out of our own heads and become present in the moment with them.

I have designed the following meditation to help you be fully present in the moment with your animal.

THE Let Go & let them MEDITATION

THIS IS A SIMPLE BUT POWERFUL MEDITATION. IT IS ABOUT BEING OPEN to letting go of your preoccupations and letting our animals take us on a trip into their world. They want us to come in, they really do. And it's a beautiful place to visit.

The best way to begin this meditation is to simply go about your normal routine, but do so while being mindful of any attempts your animal makes to engage with you. If they attempt to open up a line of communication with you through any kind of gesture (and because they don't have hands, they can get quite creative!), be it a look or stare, a bark (meow, neigh, chirp, etc.), a nose nuzzle, a tap of a paw, or their body leaning on you, rubbing up against you, or jumping on you, do the following:

- Become aware of how your animal is choosing to communicate with you.

- Slow down and stop what you are doing.

- Think of your animal's actions as if it were a human friend talking to you.

- Let go (of your own agenda) and let the animal speak to you, not just through their voice but also through their eyes and their body language.

- What are they saying? Be a good listener.

- Figure out what they're trying to tell you, what need they might have in that moment. Take your time as you try to solve their problem. It could be that they just want love and affection or to be with you, playfully or quietly. Maybe they want you to feed them or pet them or take them outside. Take the time to understand and relax into their agenda.

- Be *in the present moment* and enjoy it fully, knowing you are compassionate and caring by supporting the needs of your friend.

Having an awareness of even the tiniest of attempts of communication from your animal can have a great effect on both of you. Opening ourselves up more and more to recognize their bids at communicating with us can create endless possibilities of speaking a beautiful and unique language that exists only between the two of you.

They want us to come in, they really do. And it's a beautiful place to visit.

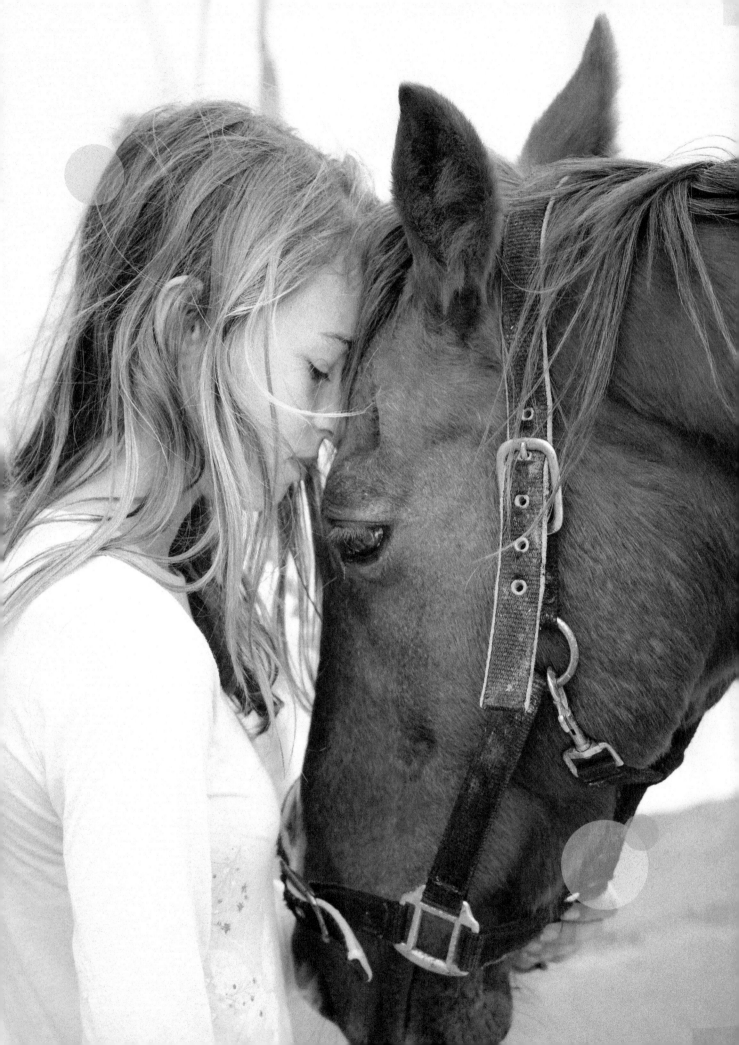

step four

Meditate

MEDITATE while sitting, walking, playing, riding, snuggling (or anything else!) with your animal

Enjoy simple things with total intensity. Just a cup of tea can be a deep meditation.

—OSHO

Meditation is really quite simple. All we have to do is embrace each experience with awareness and open our hearts fully to the present moment.

—YONGEY MINGYUR RINPOCHE

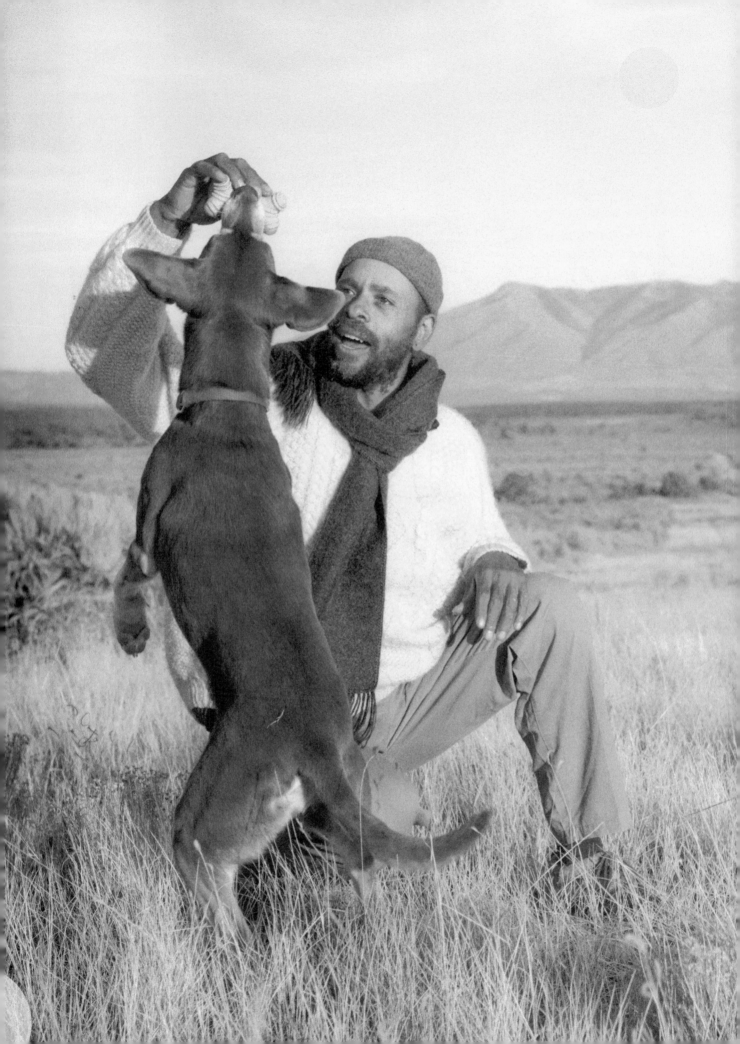

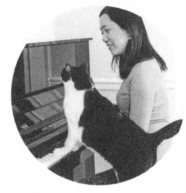

Be Your Own
GURU

MAKE UP YOUR OWN MEDITATION WITH YOUR ANIMAL COMPANIONS AND *OWN IT!*

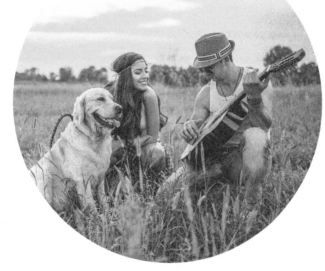

Any daily activity can be used as an opportunity for meditation.

—YONGEY MINGYUR RINPOCHE

THIS QUOTATION PRESENTS A POWERFUL CONCEPT THAT IS THE FOUN-dation for building more conscious connections with our animals through meditation: there is no one way to do it. This is an important truth to recognize, as often in life there are things we feel we must learn to do in a precise way or else we won't be doing it correctly. For many things, this is true; for others, it is not—and this includes meditation.

The word meditation comes from two Latin words: *meditari* (to think, to contemplate, to exercise the mind) and *mederi* (to heal or cure). Its Sanskrit derivation, *medha*, means wisdom. And so meditation essentially means awareness; therefore, I like to think that whatever you do with awareness can then become your meditation. Listening to music or the sound of the birds singing outside could be a meditation. Sitting under the moon could be a meditation. Walking your dog could be a meditation. As long as these activities are free from any other distraction to the mind, it is effective meditation.[17]

Throughout our lives, we store and integrate within our minds what we learn from the different people, places, things, studies, and experiences we encounter. And so, just as our teachers have become to us, we can become to ourselves: creating our own way of accumulating information and forming it into our unique way

> *Let your heart be your guide. Glean suggestions from other sources. Combine them to become your very own meditations.*

of doing things. These become our own beliefs; an amalgam of our greatest interests that have sparked our souls.

It has been said that meditation can be similar to state of mind, in that some people have the ability to produce the same brain-wave frequencies that are commonly seen in meditators *without actually meditating.*[18] This concept has great meaning to me as it suggests that we all have the ability to do this—beginning with having the curiosity and desire to explore different ideas about meditation. It asks that you recognize that a certain method of meditating is not the ultimate or only way of doing it simply because it already exists. The truth is, there are infinite possibilities for meditation that have yet to be discovered. By you! This leaves the door wide open to allow for the idea that we can create ways for ourselves and our animals to connect that are purely our own. Let your heart be your guide. Glean suggestions from other sources. Combine them to become your very own meditations.

Lastly, when it comes to meditating, I try not to allow judgment and self-criticism to become roadblocks. It is my belief that clearing your mind and connecting your heart with the heart of your beloved companion in a way that is unique to you is, at its essence, a meditation on being in the present moment—and your present moment is unique and belongs only to you! That moment has the power to change your perspective and can benefit you beyond only that snapshot in time.

Sara Lazar, a neuroscientist and study senior author at the Massachusetts General Hospital's Psychiatric Neuroimaging Research Program and a Harvard Medical

School instructor in psychology, says "Although the practice of meditation is associated with a sense of peacefulness and physical relaxation, practitioners have long claimed that meditation also provides cognitive and psychological benefits that persist throughout the day."[19]

Since I consciously introduced the practice of Meditating with Animals into my life, I have realized how many of the emotional and spiritual exchanges I've shared with my animals have lifted me up and carried me throughout my days and even into the night in my dreams. I often find that a smile will appear on my face or a sweet feeling will well up in my heart, long after the experience itself. It makes me feel softened, peaceful, comforted. It also makes me feel grateful to have animals in my life who can have such a meaningful impact on my overall well-being and state of mind.

The peaceful approach I take in my daily life affects my animal companions as well, and I discovered a very tangible way to recognize this, which I'll share with you now.

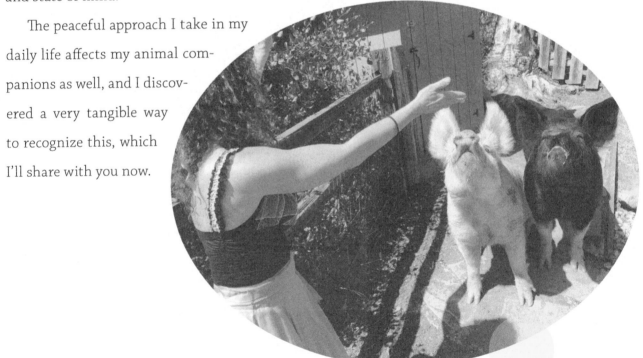

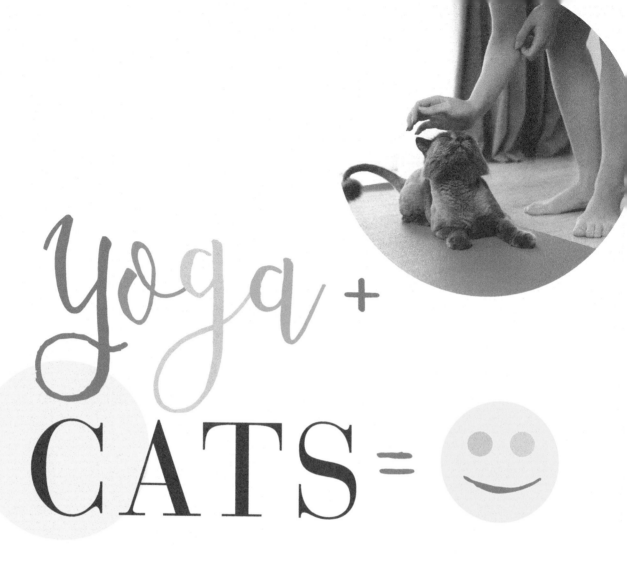

Yoga + CATS = 🙂

I PRACTICE YOGA ALMOST EVERY MORNING. FOR ME, WHETHER I DO IT for twenty, forty, or sixty minutes isn't important—it's about getting on the mat and breathing, stretching, and clearing my mind to start the day from that grounded, quiet place. I often meditate afterward to take my calm mental state a little deeper. It's been over a year since I began doing this regularly. My yoga mat is permanently out on the floor in a room in my house.

When I first started doing yoga at home, I noticed that Sylvester and Kit-Ten were wondering what I was doing. They would wander in and out of the room during my practice, unable to resist their own curious tendencies! Then they started coming in and staying for a while. I've had quite a few laughs at how they would wander around me and under me, brushing a tail or poking a wet nose on my face, or bumping or rubbing a whole body against my limbs. I've even caught Kit-Ten watching the whole "show" from various spots in the room—sometimes right up on the bench next to my mat and other times from under a piece of nearby furniture, like he's spying, which totally cracks me up. I can't help but laugh.

Not long after I'd incorporated yoga into my morning routine, I was surprised when I would come into the room and find one or both cats lying on the mat before I even got there, waiting for me to begin! And now, even if they wander away during my practice, they very often come back for what comes next: when I finish my practice I sit cross-legged on my mat and meditate. While doing this, I've had Sylvester come up on my lap. Kit-Ten likes to bump me to get my attention, which I regard as the same as a thought coming into my mind that I need to acknowledge and release. In their own ways, they each make it clear that my morning ritual is something that they also enjoy. They want it and wait for it, just as I want to do yoga and can't wait to get to my mat in the morning. It makes it an activity that we

It makes it an activity that we all benefit from. The harmonious vibrations that flow between us fill us and the space with love, tranquility, and happiness.

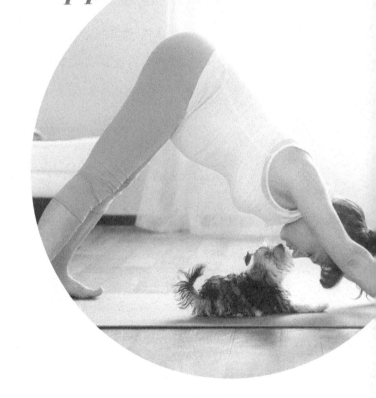

Maybe you already have an active practice ...expand into new meditation methods that include your animal companions

all benefit from. The harmonious vibrations that flow between us fill us and the space with love, tranquility, and happiness.

What I love about their eagerness to join my yoga space is that it tells me they understand this specific spot has an energy that feels good to them. Knowing that my cats like this—and that I can match and reflect their energy—has been one of the biggest insights I've discovered in relation to how Meditating with Animals works. I understand, because they have shown me, that this level of energetic connection feels good to them. It closely mirrors their natural vibration, which is why they like it so much. For my part, the feeling that I get from yoga is one that I can have in the moment and also can go back to throughout the day and tap into when I need to bring myself back to my "happy place." I do this for myself and I also do it when I am with my animal companions.

Maybe you already have an interest in meditation or an active practice. Perhaps you have even taken classes or done research that has opened doors and windows in your mind and your soul, further sparking your curiosity about meditation, healing, and relationships. Take all of what you've come to know and use it to expand into new meditation methods that include your animal companion(s). And if you haven't yet tried meditating, now is a great time to begin. It is my hope that the information I share with you in this book, along with the meditation exercises I suggest, serve to inspire you.

MY MAGICAL HORSE AND HOW WE *Meditate* TOGETHER

EVERY WEEK, I TAKE TUXEDO FOR A TRAIL RIDE OR TWO. THIS IS HIS time to relax and my time to relax with him. It's our walking/riding/talking/singing/laughing meditation—our version of what I like to call the "Everything but the Kitchen Sink" meditation (the steps for which I provide at the end of this chapter).

It starts when I jump up on Tux's back and feel my legs wrapped around his powerful body. In that moment, my feet are no longer planted on the earth and I am given a freedom to move in a way that I could not do without him beneath me. As we start walking, I pay attention to what Tux is paying attention to. I allow him to stop if he wants to smell something he finds interesting, or to see and register his surroundings if he is hesitant or curious. I create the opportunity for him and also find enjoyment in discovering what is going on in his brain. Another thing I keep in mind is that if he is worried or afraid of something, I don't push him into moving past it before he's ready to. I give him the space to figure it out first. I would never want to be forced to move past something I found scary, so it is an opportunity for me to step outside of myself and let him work through it. I give him that gift of patience, and I am rewarded with a deepened sense of trust from him.

I laugh at different things Tuxedo does on these walks and try to figure out why he's doing them. Maybe he is distracted by all the fresh green grass and is walking really fast because he remembers the exact spot up ahead where he likes to graze. Or maybe he lifts his head up high because he sees or hears something that I can't just yet, which makes me feel amazed by his sensory abilities. Sometimes he gets startled if squirrels or birds pop out of bushes or trees nearby. On other walks, there might be a horse he wants to go over and greet like a person does when they see someone they know. These little things he does make me giggle inside or sometimes just laugh out loud.

Mostly what I notice is that Tuxedo is content with it just being the two of us; he seems to feel secure and trust me, as I trust him. This confidence we have in each other allows each of us to explore and, therefore, we both benefit from the experiences that we create together. That positive energy flows between us and I remain conscious of my role as leader. The power of our connection brings me into and holds me in the present moment. When I get distracted, I just bring myself back to what Tux is doing and then I am with him fully again. That is the ebb and flow of all meditation.

We're all familiar with how our minds like to start thinking about what we should be doing rather than focusing on what we are currently doing when we're meditating, as if taking time to be with yourself is not as much of a priority. Well, I assure you, it is! I combat my mind's tendency to wander by incorporating other methods of meditation that help keep me focused during my time with Tuxedo.

One of the things I do is talk with him, the same as I would a friend or person I love. He can feel the energy I bring to him from my outside world, so I choose to share with him what's happening in my life. I call them my "Conversations with Tuxedo." I also simply tell him how much I love him and love being his mom, how I will always take care of him and how smart, handsome, brave, talented, amazing, and funny he is. I tell him the story of how I found him and that I knew he was going to be with me always. I also sing songs that I make up for him. I'm no Mariah Carey, but he doesn't care. The melodies always seem to rhythmically comingle with the sound of his hooves clip-clopping on the ground and so it feels like we're making music together.

Our voices carry our energy, and our words carry our intent. I use my voice as a tool to connect with my amazing horse by being conscious of the tone and volume in which I speak to him. I do so in a way that I would like to be spoken to by someone

When I get distracted, I just bring myself back to what Tux is doing and then I am with him fully again. That is the ebb and flow of all meditation.

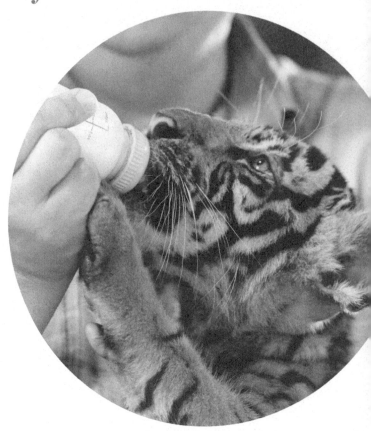

I use my voice as a tool to connect with my amazing horse by being conscious of the tone and volume in which I speak to him.

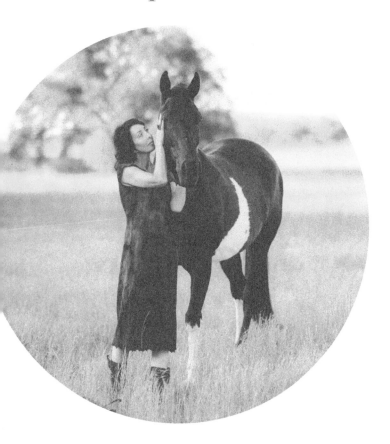

who loves and cares about me. He may not understand the language, but I feel that he understands the vibration and feelings behind my words, regardless of whether I am feeling happy, sad, or even angry. (Yes, sometimes he can make me mad or I annoy him and make him mad! It's a relationship, after all, and we are both capable of having bad days in which one of us feels tired, bossy, or impatient. One thing I know for sure is that Tux knows what I'm talking about!) I see his ears tuning in to me while I talk or sing, and this makes me smile. If I have to reprimand him in order to get him to pay attention to me and remind him I am the leader, I use a certain tone . . . and then I try not to laugh because of how quickly he responds and corrects his behavior.

Another way I meditate with Tuxedo is through touch. As I speak more about in the following chapter, when I was healing from cancer surgery, I couldn't do much, and that included riding Tux. But he still gave me a reason to get out of the house and be among my friends at the barn, out in nature, and in his healing presence. And during these

I feel that he understands the vibration and feelings behind my words.

visits, I would comb his mane, brush his body, and sponge his face with water. I would do these things quietly, sometimes never saying a word because I didn't have the energy to talk. Just being near him, touching him, smelling him, and exchanging loving energy was filling me up the like the gas tank of my car at the gas station. This fuel kept me going.

Sometimes I will just sit on the ground beneath Tuxedo's head while he eats. When he bends his neck down to reach the food, I love to close my eyes and listen to the sound of his chomping on hay and the occasional clearing of his nose through big exhales of energy that send horse nose liquid flying all over me. He'll drop pieces of hay on my head or in my lap, and I love that too. I've cried, slept, collapsed while exhausted and defeated, and also meditated in that corner of his stall many, many times. Occasionally, Tux will nudge me with his nose on my leg, hand, arm, or head, just to let me know he is there with me. I do the same. I put my hand on his head and just touch him, visualizing and sending love and deep gratitude from my heart through my fingertips to him. It is in its simplicity an incredibly beautiful and powerful connecting experience.

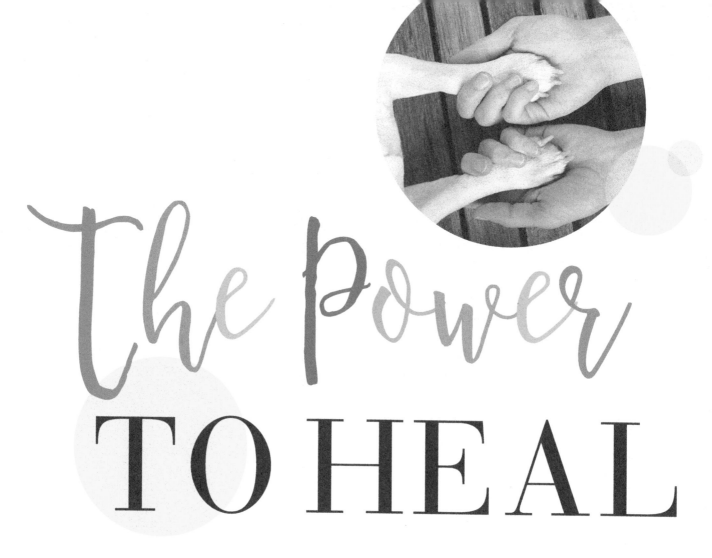

The Power
TO HEAL

BEING UNSELFCONSCIOUS ABOUT HOW I MEDITATE WITH MY ANIMALS has given me an abundance of healing gifts. I know this to be true from my own personal experience, but there is also some very exciting scientific evidence relating to the energy that comes from our hearts and how it can have an effect on the heart of another being that is near you.

The HeartMath Institute conducted a study in 1998 called *The Electricity of Touch: Detection and Measurement of Cardiac Energy Exchange Between People.* Researchers set out to determine whether the heart's electromagnetic field in one person, as measured by an electrocardiogram, could be detected and measured in another person when the pair either were sitting within about three feet of each other or holding hands.

The results of the experiment were positive: "When people touch or are in proximity, a transference of the electromagnetic energy produced by the heart occurs," the study's authors wrote. They concluded that, although additional research should be conducted, there were potential important implications raised by this research when viewed in conjunction with the success of numerous healing practices, pointing out that these practices, such as therapeutic touch, shiatsu, and Reiki, among others, "are based upon the assumption that an exchange of energy occurs to facilitate healing." They went on further to say: "While there exists scientific evidence to substantiate the physiological and psychological effects of many of these treatments, science has as yet not been able to describe a mechanism by which this putative energy exchange between individuals takes place."[20]

I know this energetic healing energy is what I experience with my animals (like I talked about in chapter 1, with Sylvester) and, even though researchers can't yet describe *how* the energy exchange occurs, I find it incredibly exciting that the scientific community is exploring the phenomenon more closely. As the HeartMath researchers point out, their study represents just one of the first successful attempts to directly measure an exchange of energy between people.

I provide steps to guide you in specific meditations customized for a certain purpose in the other chapters (learning how to be more aware of your animal, for example); and in this chapter my hope in providing the following meditation is that new ideas and pathways for meditating will be opened up and you will discover deeper connections and infinite opportunities to connect more deeply with your animal through whatever activity it is you are doing together.

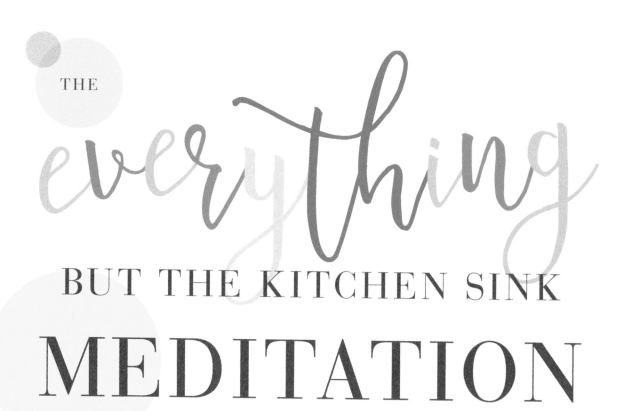

THE *everything* BUT THE KITCHEN SINK MEDITATION

THIS MEDITATION IS ABOUT TRUE CONNECTION: GENUINELY BEING with your animal, without distraction, in whatever activity the two of you are engaged in. In traditional meditation we find a quiet place and we sit, close our eyes, breathe, and go into ourselves. In this meditation, it absolutely can be sitting, any of the ways I suggest or your own inspirations. The intention is to connect our hearts with our animals. Let's begin.

What I outline below is to create the buffer between the initial act of sitting and breathing and the activity (activities!) that you choose to do once you have slowed down and come to your animal with a quieter energy, a lightened heart.

- Begin by taking a really deep breath in through your nose, followed by a really deep breath out through your mouth.

- Put your hand on your heart and continue breathing.

- Breathe in a little more deeply and breathe out, releasing any stress or tension you feel yourself holding inside. This will feel good and it will move you into a state of relaxation fairly quickly. Enjoy this mini-breathing exercise as long as you like.

- Feel your heart beating. Send gratitude to your heart for working so hard to keep you alive.

- See your heart in your mind's eye, radiating love. I like to picture it as a glowing golden sun.

- Visualize this light radiating within your body, and as you exhale send the light out to your immediate surroundings, to your animal, and then out to the world.

- Now visualize your animal's heart radiating with love, however this looks or feels to you.

- Connect your hearts by visualizing your beautiful love energy leaving your heart with your exhale and flowing into your animal's heart, filling it up. Then, on the inhale, visualize the love energy leaving your animal's heart and coming back into yours, filling you up.

- Continue the flow with each breath, returning the energy to your animal on the exhale and feeling it come back to you on the inhale. I like to imagine my animal's entire body radiating full of this loving energy.

- When you feel a sense of calm, a warm feeling, or a lightness, continue to breathe and relax for a few minutes. Heart connection established!

Now you are ready to begin your walking, talking, sitting, laying down, running, climbing, hiking, and swimming meditations! The fun part of the practice is to continue to return to the awareness through different forms of meditation and create your experience together with your hearts and minds joined as one.

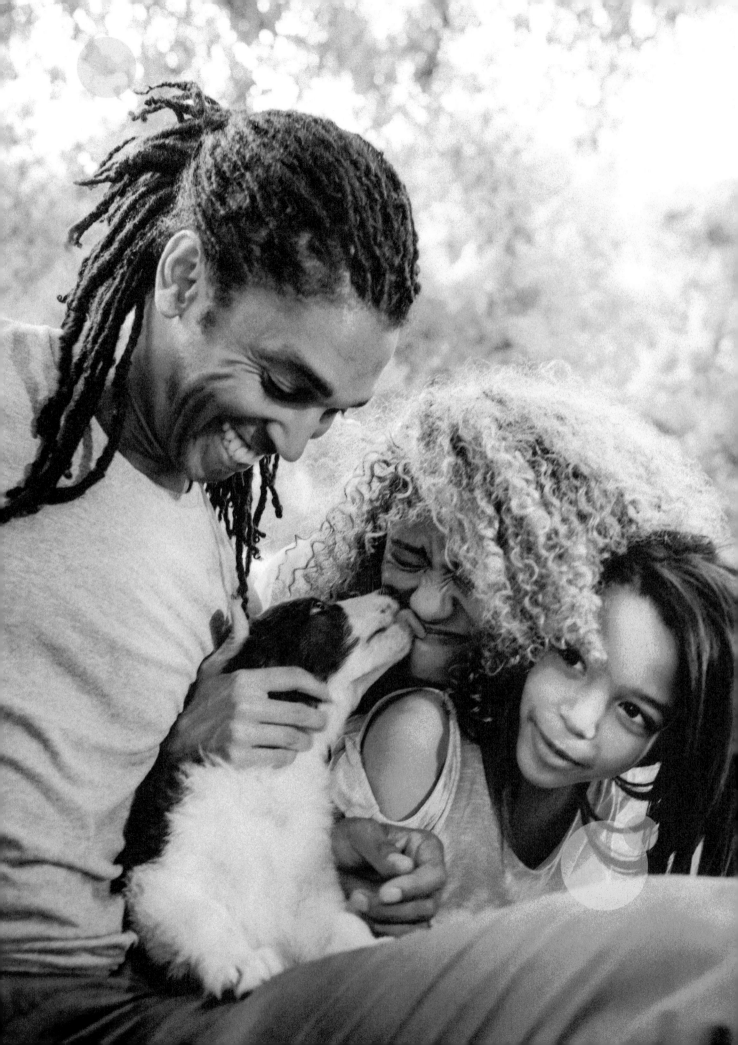

step five

Allow

ALLOWING
yourself to cherish
and savor the precious
time you have with
your animal

Let your light shine brightly, allowing others to shine their light with you.

—DAVE BLOMSTERBERG

Look at a tree, a flower, a plant. Let your awareness rest upon it. How still they are, how deeply rooted in Being. Allow nature to teach you stillness.

—ECKHART TOLLE

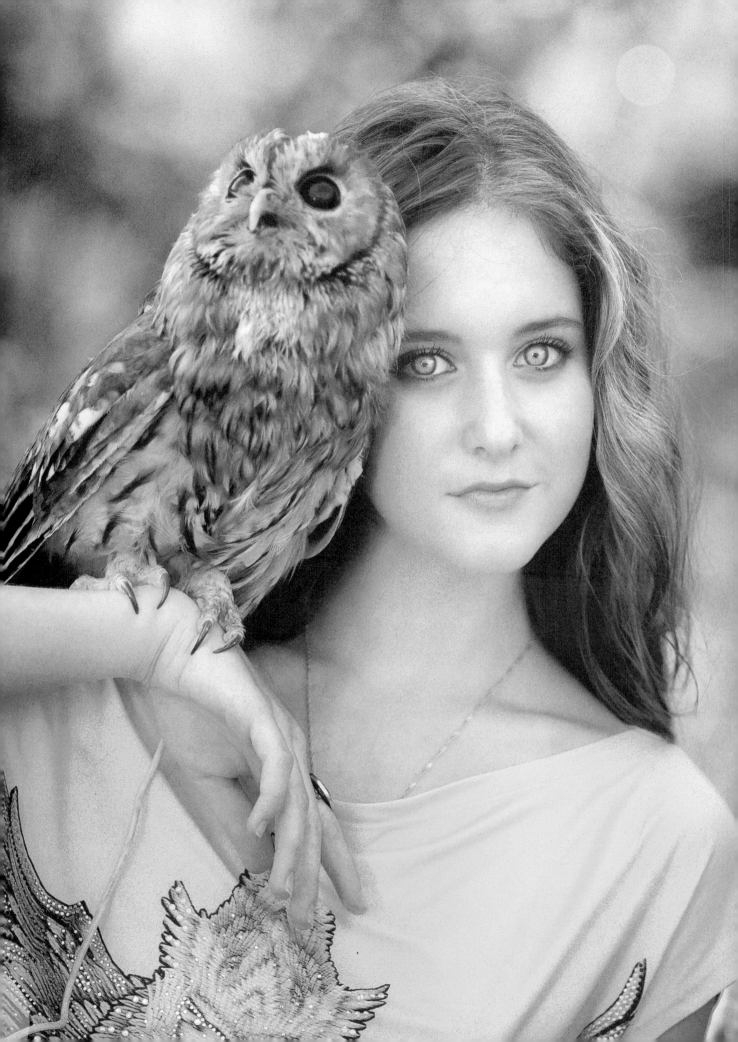

LEARNING FROM ANIMALS HOW TO SLOW DOWN AND TAKE

Better Care OF YOURSELF

THE STRESS AND STRAIN OF CONSTANT CONNECTION TO OUR OUTER world can sometimes wreak havoc with our well-being. I discovered this the hard way during what was an extremely challenging time for me, but it turned out to be an invaluable lesson that changed my life.

When I was recovering from the surgery that removed my thyroid cancer in late 2014, I was forced to take time during my healing to completely disconnect from everything so that I could allow my body to rest and recover. My mind fought a lot with this concept until I had no choice but to give in—but only because my body gave out.

I lost the ability to speak, breathe, and swallow properly for a period of eight weeks or so after the initial surgery. The cancerous tumor had been on my vocal cord, and as the tumor was being removed, it paralyzed the cord (just for good measure, as my fate would have it). This condition can be permanent because the vocal cord nerve cannot always fully repair itself, and so I required another surgery to put an implant next to the damaged cord to return my speaking voice and other functions.

I really struggled with finding a way to allow myself to rest during that time. It was a bigger undertaking than just dealing with my health situation; it was a lifetime of programming that I needed to undo. The perfectionist, the Type A personality, the workaholic, the high achiever—they were all very formidable opponents who didn't allow me much time for rest and relaxation when there was work to do, and failure was not an option. In short, my ego resisted in a very big way.

I had to wait over two very trying—and yet, as it turned out, also very enlightening—months for the second operation. It was painful to try to talk, and I couldn't catch my breath when I did. This came exactly at the time when my marriage came to a dramatic end. Screaming would have been . . . expected. Instead, it led to a major lightbulb moment for me. I had grown up in a family that screamed at each other but I came to the realization that this was not who I was; that it had been taught to me in a family environment and dynamic I never felt I truly belonged to. Because of this, I understood that the teaching could be undone. And undone it was, albeit in a way that was drastic, but I learned that there are many ways to use your voice. If you yell, people stop listening to you; they shut down. But if you are quiet, silence can be very loud. So when you choose your words carefully and say only what is necessary, those words hold more value and you are fully heard. By losing my voice for those two months I became more connected with the quiet of my own soul—and found the true and pure nature of my authentic voice.

In the weeks following the operation, my mind was so torn between wanting to feel alive and prove to myself and others that I was "OK" by being active, while at

Because I didn't want to disturb my cats, I stayed put for longer periods of time and relaxed into the protective shelter they built around my body.

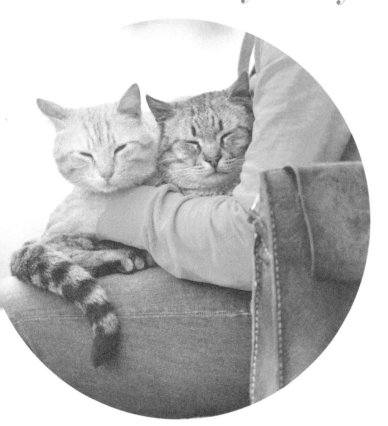

the same time I understood that my body had just been through the trauma of a surgery and so I needed to honor and support it with rest. At one point, I went so far as to write on my hand "be still, quiet, heal" to remind myself that this was my priority, my job—myself—for once and not everyone and everything else. If I wasn't well, I couldn't take care of anything. So I shifted.

Though difficult, this shift changed the way I look at my life and everything that I allow to come in it in a very positive way. I now understand the immense value of caring for myself and the effect it has on my overall well-being, and therefore the priority I must give to allowing peace, quiet, and stillness into my life. But this shift didn't come from my own abilities; my animals were my teachers.

My cats were an incredibly important part of my being still during my convalescence, when I was trying to process the death of my mother only a few weeks before, the discovery of my cancer, the resultant surgery, and the breakup of my marriage. I was traumatized and reeling from it all.

My brain couldn't digest all the new information fast enough; it would just shut down like a computer and I would have to sleep. And when I did, my cats were with me, on me, essentially part of me, whether I was in bed or on the couch. Their presence made me think once, twice, three times about getting up and being busy with some task my active mind thought was important to do. Instead, because I didn't want to disturb Sylvester, Kit-Ten, and Sophie, I stayed put for longer periods of time and relaxed into the protective shelter they built around my body. Through their presence and comfort, they did an excellent job of keeping me from getting up. Teaching by example. I have to say, keeping me still was not an easy task. Their persistence over time had a profound effect on me, even going so far as to create new neural pathways in my brain. Whenever I thought to jump up to do something, I paused and took a deep breath or two, then settled back down. Baby steps, over a period of time.

I am now not only a calmer person, I have the ability to truly relax. And because I discovered I enjoy this state of being so much, I began to practice yoga and meditation to help to continue to maintain it—a state of being very similar to that of my cats!

It was during this period of my life that I received the gift of Meditating with Animals, and it was given to me from my animals, because I saw the healing energy that was being transferred from my animals to me. Had I not accepted their invitation to allow myself to be still and quiet with them, this knowledge and appreciation would not have had the opportunity to manifest. Miracles have the room to materialize when we allow ourselves to make space in our minds and our hearts. Then we can take those miracles and share them with not only those we love and who are closest to us but also share them beyond our immediate world.

THE *Messenger*

NOT LONG BEFORE WRITING THIS BOOK, I WENT THROUGH THE PRO-cess of moving again, which for me was the fourth time in four years. This time, I was finally returning to the only place in my life that I had ever felt was truly my home. To be closer to my circle of friends, who are my chosen family. I left behind a twelve-year marriage (thirteen years together, in total), several businesses, a house, and the ghosts of many dreams—both personal and professional.

The days leading up to the latest move were very emotional. As I began to let go yet again, I remember the uncertainty I felt at the time, my mind full of questions: *What will be waiting for me? Who will I be as I re-create myself? Can I find the strength to go it alone? Will I succeed?* But one thing I didn't question was whether or not this move was the right thing to do. I knew that there was a bigger plan and that all

I had to do was stay positive and confident and follow the doors that were opening in front of me. The tears flowed as the memories poured out, making space for all the new to come in—a process I had become very used to. It was all happening so rapidly, I didn't even have time to think. A chance conversation with a friend had revealed that she purchased a house and was moving out of her rental in one month. She lived near my old neighborhood and friends. I went to look her place the next day and jumped at the chance to go "home." This is what I had asked the universe for and was quickly provided with, so it was time to act.

In the absence of fear, all is possible. This has been my biggest life lesson. However, changing patterns of thinking and behaviors is a process, and sometimes we all need reminders. This is exactly what showed up at my door one afternoon.

Making my way to my bedroom among the stacks of moving boxes, I was startled by this large silver cat with laser-green eyes and lion-like energy standing at my back door, looking in at me. I had never seen

I was startled by this large silver cat with laser-green eyes and lion-like energy

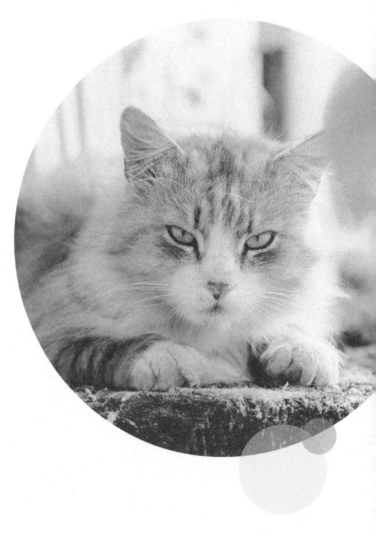

Soon I felt him conveying two words to me: powerful and independent... repeated over and over until they became part of my consciousness.

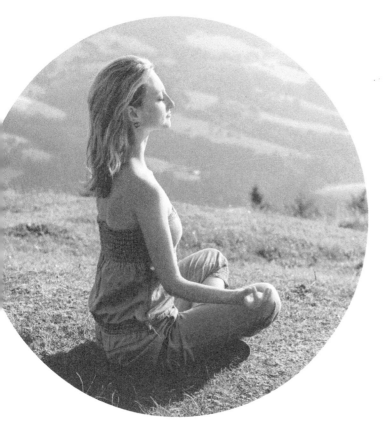

him before. He meowed to me, calling me outside. I felt compelled to be out there with him, so I opened the door and quietly slipped out, trying not to ignite the curiosity of my cats. I wanted to pet him, but for some reason, I knew that this particular meeting was not about affection and so I didn't reach down to touch him, although I sensed I could have. Instead, I was moved instinctually to sit on my outdoor couch, where I crossed my legs and laid my hands to rest on my knees. I soft-focused my eyes and began breathing deeply and meditating, going inward. The cat's eyes flashed in my mind's eye and I knew he was with me. I shuddered at the incoming energy and kept breathing.

My eyes still closed, I heard my feline visitor walking around me, and then he came to rest next to me, with his nose on my hand to let me know he was there. He pressed his body against my leg, his tail on my thigh, and crouched down beside me. I just continued to breathe. Soon I felt him conveying two words to me: *powerful* and *independent*. These words were repeated over

and over until they became part of my consciousness. I let him know that I understood by visualizing in my mind the word "yes." Without words but with my intention, I asked if he would like to receive my love in return for his gift, and he responded affirmatively. He stayed. I visualized my heart filling with a beautiful golden light and feelings of love and gratitude, and then I sent that love to his heart, his whole being.

Several minutes passed as we sat with big love energy moving back and forth and all around us. Then, when he was finished, he jumped off the couch, walked across the yard, and was gone. My heart was racing. He was a messenger who had brought me exactly what I needed to hear in that moment. His power and independence were undeniable from the very first second I locked eyes with him, and he wanted me to see that in myself. By allowing him the freedom to deliver his message, I was able to receive it and use it as an important and necessary reminder as I boldly entered into the newest chapter of my life.

I now offer you the following meditation, which will help you, through the use of conscious breathing, to focus on the presence of your animal, and in doing so, become aware of and allow in any wisdom they may have to share with you.

DON'T HOLD YOUR *Breath* MEDITATION

THE FOUR-SEVEN-EIGHT BREATH TECHNIQUE IS ONE OF MY FAVORITE meditation practices because it's very simple and the counting keeps me engaged. I also like that it doesn't require a lot of time and you can do it anywhere. The counting of breath calms the nervous system, acting as a natural tranquilizer.[21]

- Relax in a comfortable seated position on the floor, on a bed, or on a couch or in a chair, with your hands resting on your knees and your palms facing up or down.

- Close your eyes.

- Exhale, sending all of your breath out of your mouth while making a *whooshing* sound.

- Close your mouth and inhale through your nose for a count of **four**.

- Hold your breath for a count of **seven**.

- Exhale, sending all of your breath out of your mouth for a count of **eight**.

- After a few rounds, you should start to feel a sense of relaxation come over you.

- Let your shoulders drop down to further relax and let go. This is my favorite part because the tension will leave your body. You don't feel how tense you really are until you release your shoulders!

- Now, as you continue to breathe, visualize your heart being like a sun—a golden ball—warm and glowing. Focus on this beautiful feeling for several more inhales and exhales.

- At this point, I like to turn my palms face up and, on my next exhale, send the warm glowing feeling of love I have created in my heart, outward, to my animal's heart, asking if they would like to join me in this loving, peaceful space.

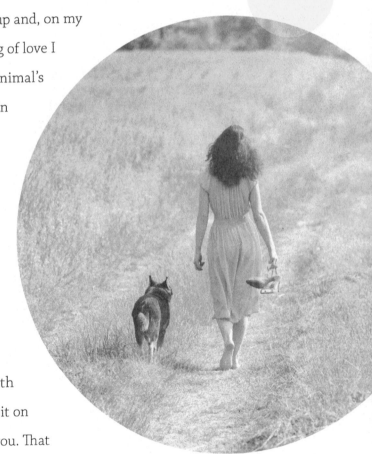

- I do this by visualizing a beautiful path between my heart and my animal's heart. In my mind, I ask them if they would like to meet and join me on this path. The key is that your calmness and loving intent is your invitation that allows your animal the freedom to choose to join you.

- Sometimes your animal is already there with you, physically or energetically. They may sit on you, sit near you, or walk away or around you. That doesn't mean they aren't enjoying your calm and peaceful vibe. They have their own way of enjoying it and you.

- Once you are connected with your animal, just continue to breathe in and out love, as you visualize the details of the beautiful pathway you imagined sharing with your animal, and enjoy the tranquil vision you have created for them and with them. Is there grass? Are there flowers, trees, rocks? Is the path long and winding? Narrow or wide? You simply could be sitting in the warm sun-filled rays of love light you have sent out to them. It's your vision in the moment.

- Continue sharing that loving energy just being in this "other world" of peaceful-ness and beauty until you or your animal are done. The time is not important; the exercise of intention, visualization, connectivity, and calm are.

- Take five minutes or more anytime you feel it would benefit you (both) to shift into a lower gear. This stress-free time is healing and beneficial for both of you.

I like to end this meditation by thanking my animal for being all of who they are and for all the wonderful things they bring into my life.

Feelings come and go like clouds in a windy sky. Conscious breathing is my anchor.

—THICH NHAT HANH

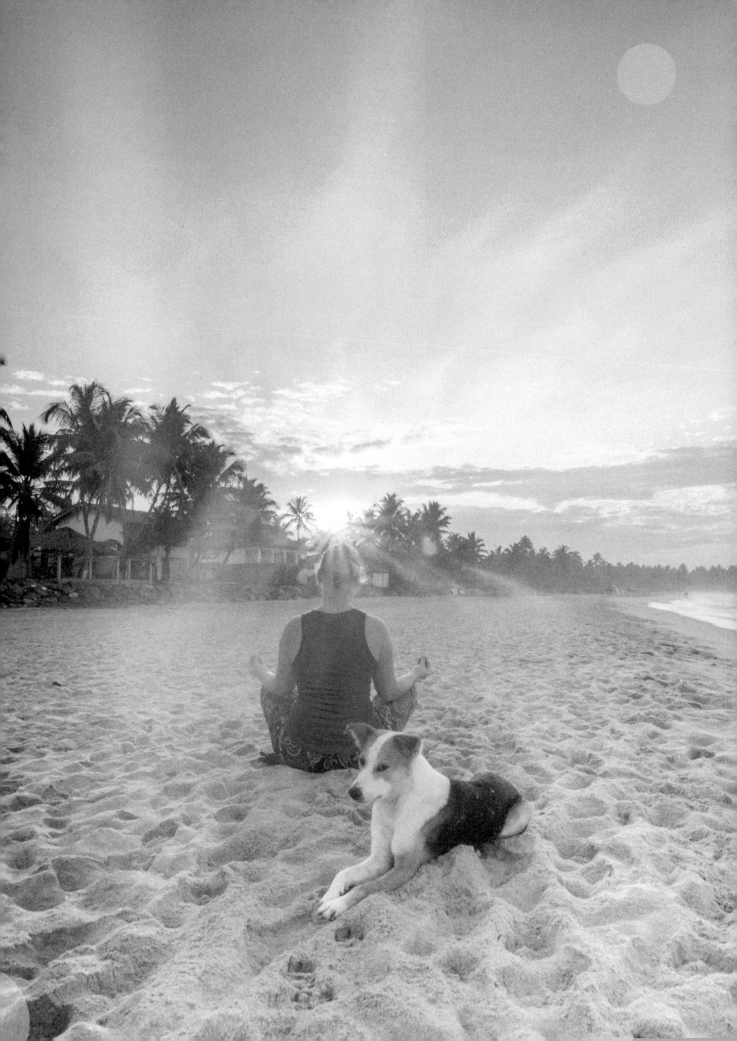

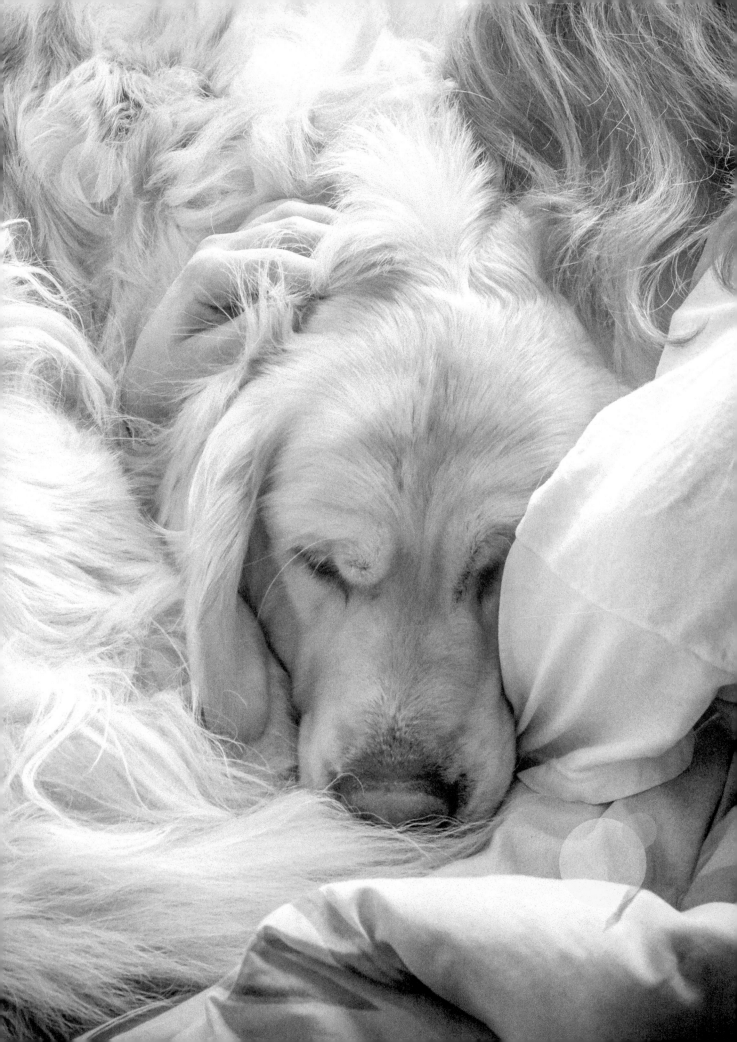

step six

Love

recognizing the
power of **LOVING**
and the human-
animal bond

Love cures people, both the ones who give it and the ones who receive it.

—DR. KARL MENNINGER

Friendship is the purest love. It is the highest form of love where nothing is asked for, no condition, where one simply enjoys giving.

—OSHO

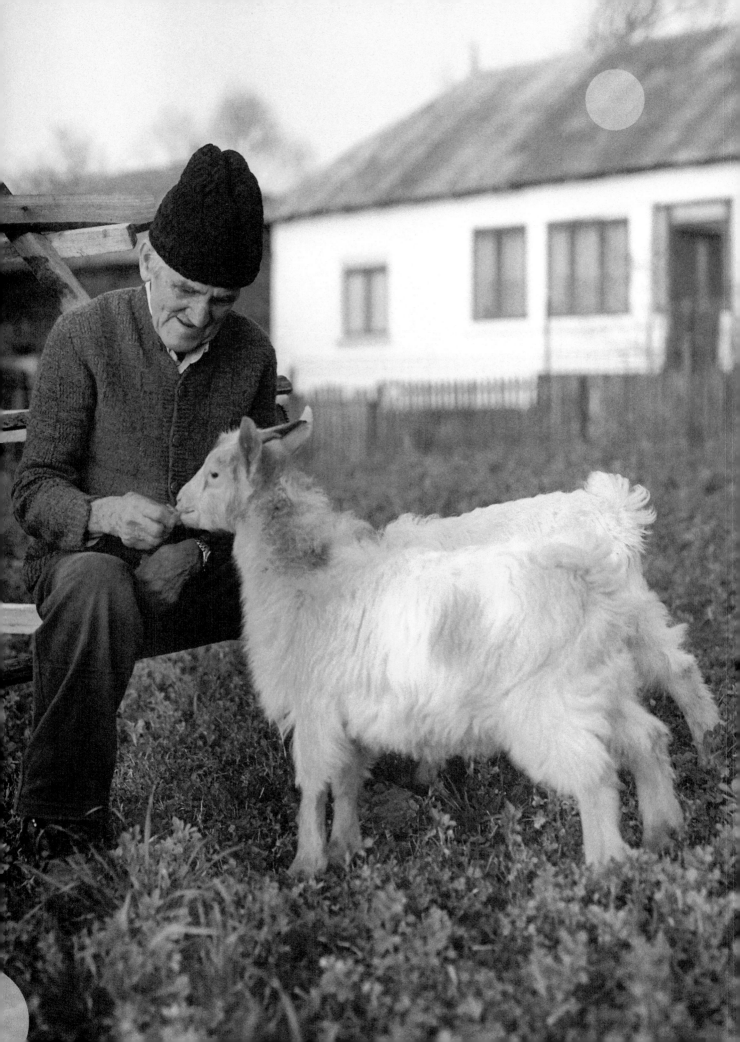

the Energy
OF LOVE

OUR UNIVERSE AND OUR PLANET ARE MADE OF ENERGY—EVERYTHING
that we see is energy. We are made of energy, and so is everything around us: animals, plants, minerals, places, and even objects. As Albert Einstein put it, "Everything is a vibration." Your "vibe" is one way of describing your overall state of being, which is made up of different energy levels: physical, mental, emotional, and spiritual. Each of these levels has a vibrational frequency, which combines to create your overall vibration of being. For example, think about how you feel when you are giving or receiving love. This uplifting energy raises your vibration and as you radiate this energy out into the world, others will pick up on it and be attracted to your positive life force.[22]

Susan Wagner is an Integrative Medicine Doctor at MedVet Columbus who is a respected veterinary neurologist and a pioneer in the area of the human–animal bond. What I admire about her work is that it blends science, spirituality, and the wisdom of the animal kingdom. In researching Dr. Wagner's work, I learned some very relevant and meaningful things about how sensitive animals are and how they experience energy, including the following insight:

We can choose to more consciously provide them with surroundings that are as full of positive, loving vibrations as possible

- Animals serve many roles when it comes to energy and the planet. Their energy fields are far more expansive than ours—a dog's energy field is approximately 10 times that of a human's. A horse's field will encompass a large arena and a cat's will fill an entire property.

- Animals function from instinct, which is just another word for energy. In addition to their heightened senses of sight, hearing, and smell, they sense what is all around them. It is as if they have a radar.[23]

Our animal companions are using their instincts to navigate us and our energy when they are with us.

In becoming aware of the constant energetic exchanges we are having with them, we can then choose to more consciously provide them with surroundings that are as full of positive, loving vibrations as possible for the highest benefit to all of our health and well-being.

The complex energetic bonds we have with the animals that are in our lives can

Observing how our animals love us unconditionally can open our hearts to being more compassionate and more aware of how we love.

create seemingly inexplicable interactions that, if looked at more closely, seem to make perfect sense.

Dr. Wagner tells her clients that whatever is going on with someone's state of being, it can't be hidden from an animal—meaning that animals sense our energy fields. So while we may not yet be *consciously* aware of or know what is happening within our bodies, like symptoms of an illness or outward signs of stress, our energy fields are already telling a story to our animals because they read them by instinct.

Subsequently, Dr. Wagner explains to her clients that taking good care of themselves is one of the best things they can do for their animal companions and an excellent form of veterinary preventive medicine.[24] When I learned of this, it reminded me of how my sweet Sophie was diagnosed with hyperthyroidism. Thankfully, she underwent radioactive iodine treatment and went on living a healthy life for many years. It was about two years after her diagnosis that my thyroid cancer was discovered and I, too, underwent radioactive

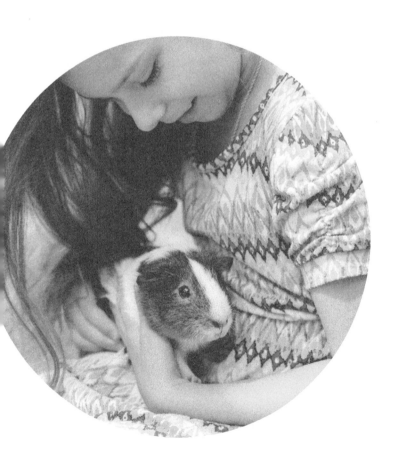

iodine treatment. Could it be that Sophie had been absorbing my illness in an act of selfless compassion? That with her excessive talking she was trying to communicate this to me? Throughout my recovery, Sophie rarely left my side and provided me with a seemingly endless amount of healing energy and support with her constant, loving presence. Was it just a coincidence, or was there more to it?

Another story that comes to mind is one my friend Krista told me, of how a cat was "gifted" to her and her boyfriend because the owner was moving and couldn't have an animal where she would be living. At first Krista wasn't overly excited about the idea. On Day One, the two just kind of checked each other out. On Day Two, they fell in love. On Day Three, Skipper was laying on her chest, purring. Not long after that, Krista was diagnosed with breast cancer. Coincidence? After her surgery, Skipper's love and their bond became an important part of her life and healing journey.

The most documented story is that of Oscar the Cat who resides on the third floor of Steere House Nursing and Rehabilitation Center in Providence, Rhode Island. Oscar has the ability to recognize when a patient is close to death and will stay near them. What is so remarkable about this is that Oscar is performing several loving and compassionate acts with his instinctual gifts. He provides companionship to the patient during their final hours, allows the staff to increase hospice services by keeping patients as comfortable as possible, and gives the staff sufficient time to notify the family. Oscar was written about in the *New England Journal of Medicine* (and later in the book *Making Rounds with Oscar: The Extraordinary Gift of an Ordinary Cat*) by David Dosa, MD, MPH a practicing geriatrician and health services researcher at Brown University.[25]

These are just a few examples of the ways that demonstrate just how closely in tune animals are with the humans around them and thus how they show their love.

There's no question that the energy of love—unconditional love—is of great importance for all of us. Professor Mario Beauregard of Montreal University's Neuroscience Research Center conducted a study on this subject. According to him, "Unconditional love, extended to others without exception, is considered to be one of the highest expressions of spirituality." Beauregard's discoveries indicated that some of the areas of the brain that were stimulated when experiencing unconditional love were also involved in the release of dopamine, the chemical that helps control the brain's reward and pleasure centers. In his research, Beauregard wrote: "The rewarding nature of unconditional love facilitates the creation of strong emotional links. Such robust bonds may critically contribute to the survival of the human species."[26]

When it comes to bonds, the loving bond we experience with our animal companions is profound, as noted above. Our animals show us unconditional love in its purest form. They don't judge us—not our failures, our shortcomings, our anger, our sadness, our depression, our illness, our grief, our inability to cope, our emotions, or even our excitement, silliness, or anything else for that matter. They love us for exactly who we are. We are free to be our authentic selves with them.

For animals, love is not given or taken, held or desired; it is a state of being that just is. By contrast, human love often comes from need and conditions. Our animal companions show us how to love more naturally, without the conditions we place on ourselves as humans. Observing how our animals love us unconditionally can open our hearts to being more compassionate and more aware of how we love not only them but also the other people in our lives. So, loving unconditionally is an exercise we can practice. Think of it like an emotional muscle. When used regularly, our capacity to love grows and expands. Animals allow us on a daily basis to exercise our love, and in turn, we all benefit from the remarkable and positive effects of feeling this uplifted energy.

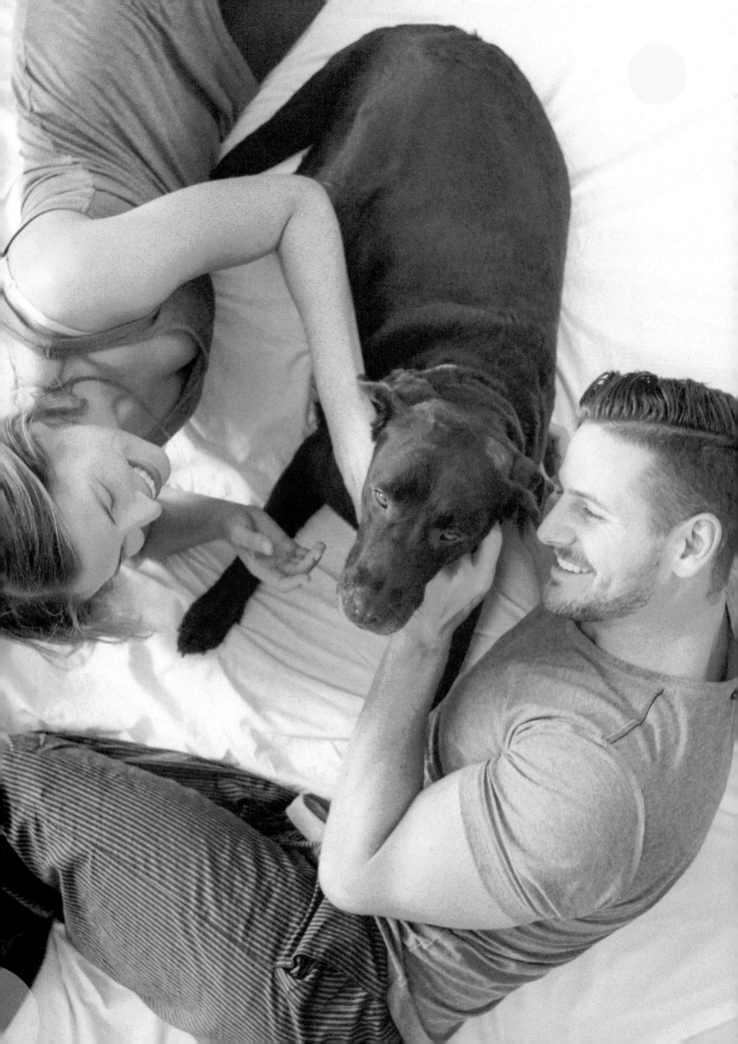

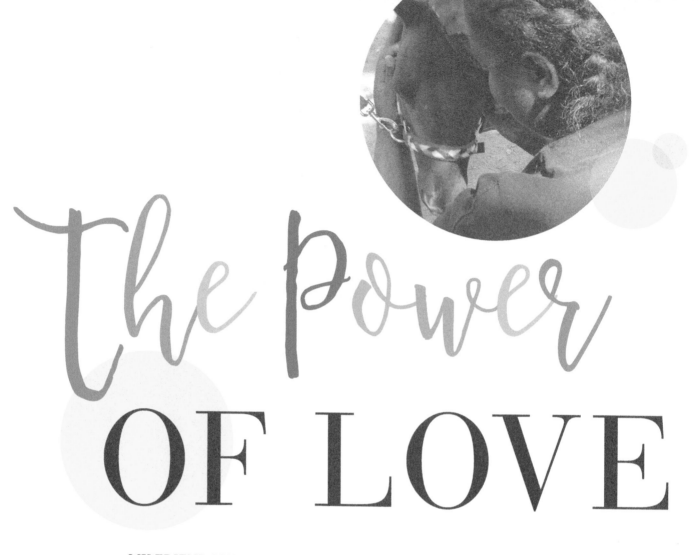

The Power
OF LOVE

MY FRIEND VICTORIA IS A REMARKABLE WOMAN WHO HAS TAKEN ON many roles, including wife, mother, artist, equestrian, and philanthropist. She is blessed with a heart that is so overflowing with love that she was moved to create a way to be able to share this love. It began with one miniature horse, a beautiful black-and-white mare named Pearl, whom she trained to be a therapy horse.

Pearl and Victoria visit the patients at the veterans hospital in Los Angeles on a weekly basis. Convincing the hospital administrators that a horse could be trained in this way was not a simple task, but they were open to the idea and it wasn't long before the doctors and staff noticed the uplifting effect Pearl had on the patients. With each new week, the requests for visits expanded to all of the hospital floors, including the psychiatric ward, where Pearl's presence drew the patients to her. Some wanted to simply touch her or gently pet her; others liked to brush her mane and tail, talk to her, or watch her perform some of the many fun tricks she has learned, like standing up on her back legs when given a "Hi ho silver!" command, smiling when asked, or playing a tune on a mini keyboard. All of these things bring the patients into Pearl's energy and release them from depression, isolation, anxiety—any negative feelings they may have been experiencing in the moments prior.

As Victoria's understanding of how horses can touch, heal, and change lives grew, so did her desire to do more. She now has seven miniature therapy horses that she has trained to visit those who are in need of these kinds of powerful interactions. Victoria, her horses, and volunteers now visit the Los Angeles and Pasadena Ronald McDonald Houses and the Greater Los Angeles Veterans Affairs Hospitals, are a part of the Los Angeles Mayor's Crisis Response Team, and are volunteers with the Los Angeles County Sheriff's Department. They also touch the lives of those at the Children's Hospital Los Angeles, Camp Gung-Ho (Children's Burn Foundation), Stewart House, UCLA Rape Center, A Place Called Home in South Central Los Angeles, Camp Erin (Our House Grief Support Center), and Maryvale Orphanage.

The experience that a person can share with one of these special horses can be incredibly powerful and have a lasting effect on their day or even their life. One of Victoria's most touching stories (and there are so many) involves one with her and Pearl. I'll share it with you now.

Victoria had received a call from the head nurse of the hospice at the Sepulveda veterans hospital on behalf of an elderly patient whom Victoria and Pearl had visited there previously. The nurse told Victoria that the patient's last request was

The experience that a person can share with these special horses can be incredibly powerful and have a lasting effect on their day or even their life.

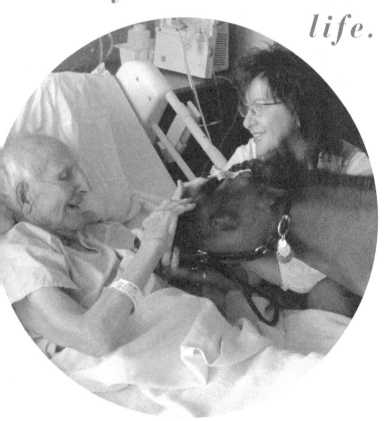

to see Pearl one more time. She said he had a few weeks yet to live, but Victoria felt an urgency and was there within a few days.

During their visit, the gentleman slipped in and out of consciousness. In his conscious moments, he shared the story of his early childhood when he had been taken in by a family who lived on a farm in Germany. He had wonderful memories of being with the horses and caring for them there. Pearl visiting him brought that beautiful reflection back into his life, and he felt a real connection with her. The bed was lowered so Pearl could be close to the dying man. He held Pearl's face and explained to Victoria how to care for her—to brush her every day and love her. He passed away only a few days after their visit, leaving Victoria feeling as if Pearl had helped him to transition.

Victoria has said the following about how she came to do what she does: "I used to pretend I was a horse when I was a child in Wisconsin. As an artist, I painted animals all my life, always feeling as if I was the animal in the painting—like they were self-portraits. It was my way of viewing and making sense out of the world. Animals have been the common thread throughout my life that grounded, calmed, and connected me to myself. Now with these miniature therapy horses, I am able to help others feel a sense of normalcy, comfort, and joy in many different types of crisis situations."[27]

There is no question in my mind that Victoria and her miniature therapy horses are vessels of love and the work they do is very important. Victoria creates the opportunities for her animals to use their natural abilities along with their training to touch hearts and heal lives. It is nothing short of astonishing to see how her sweet animal angels have the ability to know exactly what a person needs and adjust their energy and reactions instinctively. When the person the horses are interacting with experiences joy, pleasure, appreciation, and love, those feelings and that energy are returned to the horses in a reciprocal exchange.

This phenomenon is best explained by Dr. Marty Becker, "America's Veterinarian," who calls it the "love loop." As he puts it, "The love loop is a close, familiar, affectionate, loving interaction, which is intimacy. The nature/nurture factors release endocrine hormones and [those hormones control] the immune system. This bond is a simple, surefire, powerful healing power."[28]

The following story shows just how powerful this bond and its healing benefits can be.

MAYAN KEEPER OF TIME:
the great
STRIPED CAT

I WAS SO FORTUNATE TO HAVE ONE OF "THE GREATS" DURING MY TIME living in Mexico. He basically came with the home my (then) husband and I rented there. The day we arrived to move in, there was nothing in the house but a half-empty bag of dry food left out on a table, and so I assumed somebody would be showing up for a feeding at some point. A day or two went by and sure enough, arrive he did. He was cool. Magic; striped; from the jungle we lived in. I fed him and he showed up every day after. We named him Striped Cat.

We worked from home at the time, in a bedroom-turned-office on the second floor of the house. Striped Cat would jump up on the roof of our car, then climb up to the top of the carport, then jump to the balcony outside where we were working, and meow to get in. I never understood how he knew how to get to us there, but he did. He became part of our family.

After a visit to the vet one day for some dental work, they had Striped Cat's blood-work done as is routine. The results showed that he had both feline leukemia and feline immunodeficiency virus (a.k.a. cat AIDS), which is extremely common among the feral cat population in Mexico. His prognosis wasn't good for the long term—actually, not even for the short term. In Mexico they usually put cats to sleep who are living outside with these diseases, to prevent the diseases from being spread through fighting (via saliva and blood) and the animals from suffering a horrible death. But this cat was incredibly special and we loved him dearly, so although it was recommended, we just could not put him down. He had a reason for being and a life to live with us—he had made this very clear. We decided to keep him safe indoors and see what happened.

Our love affair with Striped Cat continued on a grand scale. I call him the "Mayan Keeper of Time" because he was with us for our epic life chapter in Mexico of eight years, then moved with us to California, where he was with us for almost four years

This cat was incredibly special and we loved him dearly....He had a reason for being and a life to live with us.

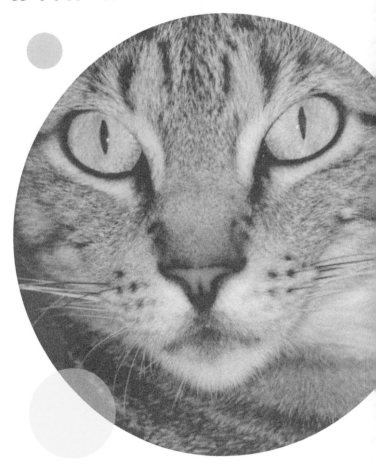

I saw him only as the little guy I met that day who was so vibrant— a real jungle cat.

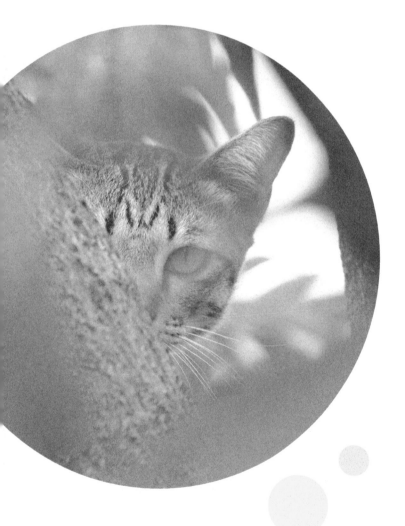

more. The doctors couldn't believe he was living as long as he was with his precarious health. We said he ran on love, and I believe with all my heart that it is why he lived so long. We worshiped and adored him, and he knew how special he was to us and his animal companions—Sophie, Sylvester, and Beauty School, our other cats. Our worlds revolved around him. We were very aware that every moment we had with him was valuable. I never looked at him as if he was sick; I never sent that energy to him. I saw him only as the little guy I met that day who was so vibrant—a real jungle cat. I didn't do this because I was in denial but because I wanted to support him with positive energy, thoughts, and feelings from my heart to his heart, not reflect back what I knew or saw with my eyes.

It was so hard to let him go when his health finally failed. I wanted more moments. He was nothing short of a miracle to the doctors, but it wasn't a miracle to me: it was pure unconditional love that had allowed him to thrive against all odds. But it wasn't until later that I realized that

Letting him go was also loving him

letting him go was also loving him. I was holding on to him for me at the end because I didn't want his life to end. And he was holding on *for* me because he knew I wasn't ready to say goodbye and I needed him still. I wish I could say his exit had been without suffering, but when you try everything possible to hold on to every last speck of life, all you are increasing is the quantity of days, not the quality. I saw this afterward when it was too late, and it is a lesson that I will never have to learn again.

Striped Cat taught me about grace, selflessness, and the human–animal bond of hearts. He taught me that when it comes to love, sometimes you just have to honor the time you had, let go, and trust that it is the best decision you can make. That you will survive without it in its current form and that the energy of the relationship and the memories you can still so clearly see, feel, taste, and even smell don't leave along with the body. The spirit remains as part of you.

I miss him every day, but I am so grateful for our time together, and I share what I learned through his teachings with others. Most recently I was able to share this wisdom with my friend Deane, who was dealing with the illness of her cherished animal companion. Cassie was an older horse and had lived a full, wonderful life with Deane

I am forever grateful for the gift that Striped Cat gave me. It enables me to share what I've learned with others and help them see the bigger picture.

as her guardian, riding trails and being pampered and adored. But sadly, Cassie was now suffering from cancer and it had gotten to the point where her body could no longer keep up the fight. Her tumors on the outside were visibly worsening, she had a fever and was fighting an infection that several rounds of antibiotics couldn't cure.

I watched my friend with awe and compassion as her tireless, loving, kind, and selfless soul did everything possible to make Cassie comfortable and try to help her fight the disease. I also saw Cassie holding on for Deane—mirroring her owner with her tireless, loving, kind, and selfless soul in return. I learned so much from just observing the two of them during the weeks that this unfolded. I knew in my heart that Cassie was ready to let go, but she couldn't because Deane wasn't ready.

One quiet afternoon at the barn, Deane and I sat on a couple bales of hay in the stillness of the feed room. We talked about the situation. We discussed the veterinarian's opinions yet lack of definitive suggested action steps about what to do. We agreed that it was up to Deane to decide how much longer she wanted to fight for Cassie's life. I shared with her my belief that she already had the answer in her heart, she just needed to see it from another perspective: Cassie was suffering but was holding on until Deane was ready to let go. I shared with her my story about Striped Cat and how I had known he couldn't fight anymore but I couldn't bring myself to let him go. I told her how, looking back, I realized that I couldn't prevent the inevitable and that I could have spared him some of the suffering in his final weeks or even days if I had said goodbye sooner. I'm crying as I write these words because this was such a difficult lesson to learn and live with, and I still miss him and regret not being able to see what was right in front of me. I am forever grateful for the gift that Striped Cat and this experience gave me, though. It enables me to share what I've learned with others and help them see the bigger picture— something that is so difficult to do when all we want in the moment is for every second of time we have left with our precious animals to go on forever.

Early one morning, not too long after we spoke, Deane let Cassie go when she was ready. It was brave and gracious and it honored Cassie for all she gave during their time together. My friend gave Cassie dignity in this choice by letting her rest in peace and not having to fight or be in pain any longer. I will always honor her for this incredible act of compassion.

The following meditation will show you how to create that special human-animal bond through giving and receiving of love with abandon and joy, making the most of each precious moment you have together.

THE
ALL YOU NEED
Is Love
MEDITATION

I ABSOLUTELY LOVE THIS MEDITATION! I PROBABLY DO THIS ONE THE most often, even combining it with other meditations, because it is so simple and makes me feel happy and full of love as soon as I begin to do it.

The mantra for this meditation is simply *love*. You will be repeating "Love . . . Love . . . Love." I prefer this as a liberal sitting meditation, which means you can traditionally sit or lie down or even play an instrument and sing the mantra or a song if you like. The objective is to focus and gather the feelings of love so that you can really quiet your mind and body and focus on creating the vibration of love for you and for your animal.

You could be brushing your dog, cat, horse, or hamster; petting your lizard, snake, or bird; watching your fish swim. Remember, we're not being formal here! If your animal companion is near you, you are ready.

- Close your eyes. Begin breathing.

- After a few deep in and out breaths, when you have relaxed into your body, just begin to breathe in the word *love* and breathe out the word *love* with the intention flowing from your heart to your animal's heart in gratitude for him or her being in your life and all the gifts he or she gives you. For example, your intention could be that you are returning healing and support to your animal to fill them up for all they have given you.

- Imagine every cell in your body illuminated as the total embodiment of the word *love*.

- You can silently repeat "love" over and over in your mind, sending the feeling to your animal.

- You can chant the word "love" out loud, envisioning love surrounding both of you.

- You can make up a silly song or glorious serenade about how much or why you love your animal (depending on your skills or personality—mine are usually silly but meaningful and heartfelt!) and sing your heart out to their heart with the intention of love.

- You can continue putting your hand on them or holding them close to you, just cradling them with the intention of having them receive your love.

- Imagine every cell of your animal's body illuminated as the total embodiment of the word *love*.

- When you feel complete, allow this feeling that you have created to linger for as long as possible.

There can be a joyful, happy, peaceful, buzzing, light feeling created by calling in all this love energy, so enjoy this, knowing that your animal is feeling it too!

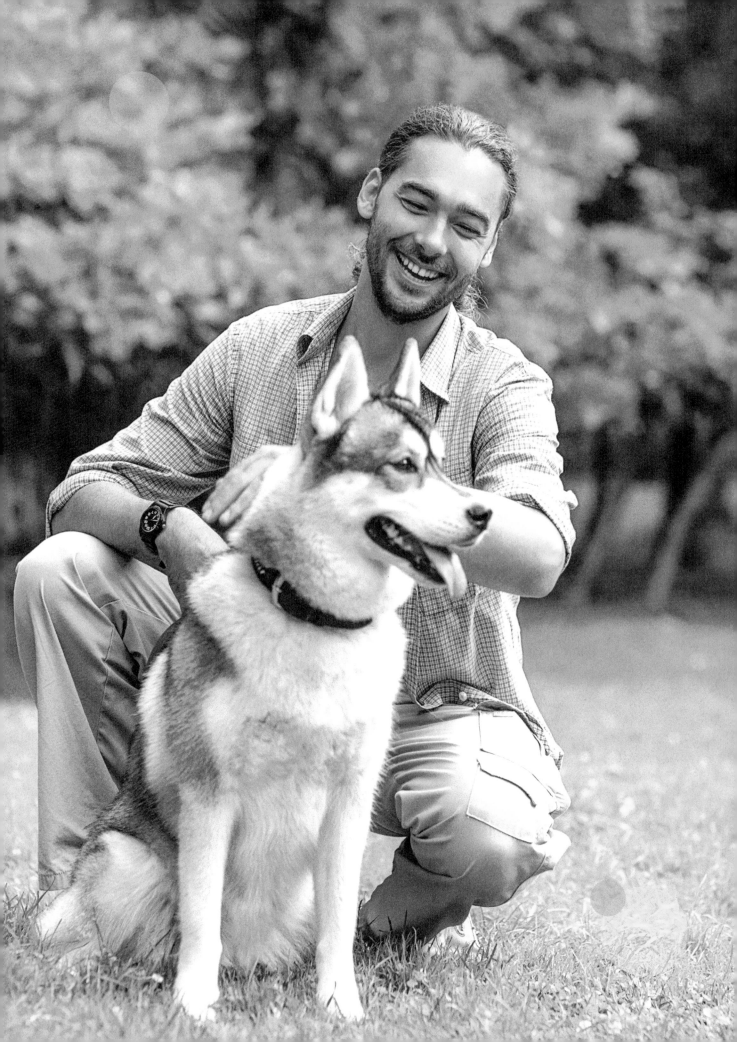

step seven

Stay

STAYING in the stillness of the moment and experiencing the magic

Study nature.
Love nature.
Stay close to nature.
It will never fail you.

—FRANK LLOYD WRIGHT

Patience is about understanding the right moment for action and the right moment for stillness.

—ALBERTO VILLOLDO

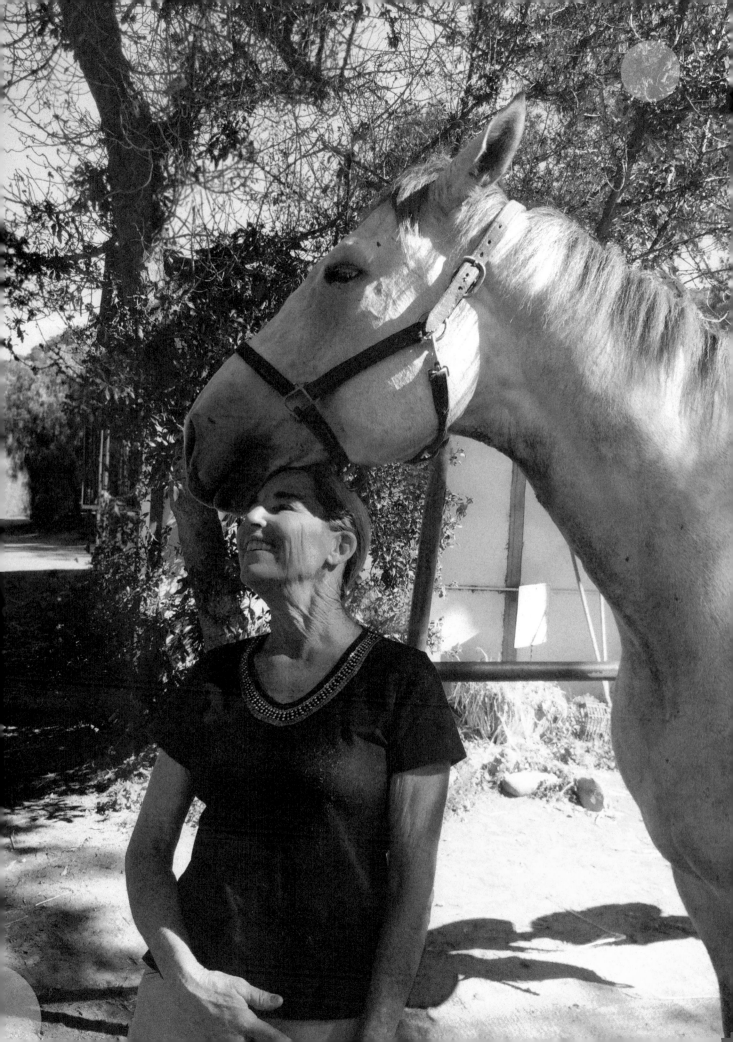

Practicing STILLNESS

QUIET IS MORE THAN JUST THE ABSENCE OF SOUND. IT GOES MUCH deeper . . . into a stillness that one can experience while hiking in the mountains or gazing at a piece of artwork in a museum or gallery. Being brought into stillness can lift your spirits and calm your mind. Michael Hunter, MD, of the University of Sheffield's Department of Neuroscience, says, "Tranquility is a state of calmness and reflection, which is restorative compared with the stressful effects of sustained attention in day-to-day life."[29]

Quiet is the doorway, an invitation to experience tranquility, healing, and restoration, and it creates real physical benefits. The mind–body connection that becomes established has been shown to relax muscles, lower anxiety and pain, and enhance a person's overall sense of well-being. In fact, all spiritual disciplines embrace quiet as the pathway to the divine. The methods may differ in how you get there, be it through silent meditation, prayer, chants, or visual imagery, but the destination is the same.[30]

Many of the people I know, including myself, have a difficult time being still. One reason for this is simply that the world is an exciting place with so many things to do, but we have limited time and so we want to make the most of every minute. Another reason is that in order to provide and care for ourselves and our families, there are not enough hours in the day to work and accomplish every task at hand. Avoidance of feelings of loneliness, anxiety, grief, sadness, pain, loss or suffering from life challenges and situations can also be a big reason. If you keep moving and your mind is busy, then there isn't any space for painful or uncomfortable thoughts or emotions to enter. In this way being busy is a well-disguised form of self-protection.

Eckhart Tolle writes so beautifully about stillness. In fact, he wrote an entire book on the topic, entitled *Stillness Speaks*. In it, he says the following:

> *When you look at a tree and perceive its stillness, you become still yourself. You connect with it at a very deep level. You feel a oneness with whatever you perceive in and through stillness. Feeling the oneness of yourself with all things is true love.*[31]

I will never forget when I experienced true stillness, in a way that was so powerful I felt transported to another place and time. I almost couldn't comprehend what was . . . *not* happening around me.

After a hike up to the top of a mountain in New Mexico, I sat down on a rock to rest. I looked around at the greatness surrounding me in every direction and

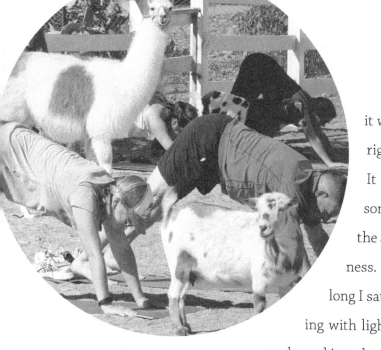

it was almost too much to take in. It didn't happen right away, but then it hit me. Hard. It hurt my ears. It was deafening silence. I almost wanted to hear something to make it stop. My brain didn't compute the absence of sound. I was in awe. Then I was in stillness. Stunning, beautiful stillness. I don't know how long I sat there taking it in. It filled me up and I was buzzing with lightness of being. As the stillness embraced me, I embraced it and we became one.

The Animal Method helps you achieve stillness by connecting with your animal, thereby quieting your mind. Choose any (or all!) of the meditations offered within these pages to do so. Once you've achieved stillness, the next step—staying—involves lingering in that experience with your animal and benefitting together from sharing the stillness.

Nature and animals have always been the key drivers for my desire to be still. The moments shared are so special that it is almost like a spell I don't want to break. When you are experiencing something magical—which connection to animals and nature absolutely can be—it is in these moments you almost have the ability to not only find stillness in yourself but also to find stillness in time. There is poetry in stillness, and it is yours to write.

The following little story was one I was happy to be able to write about.

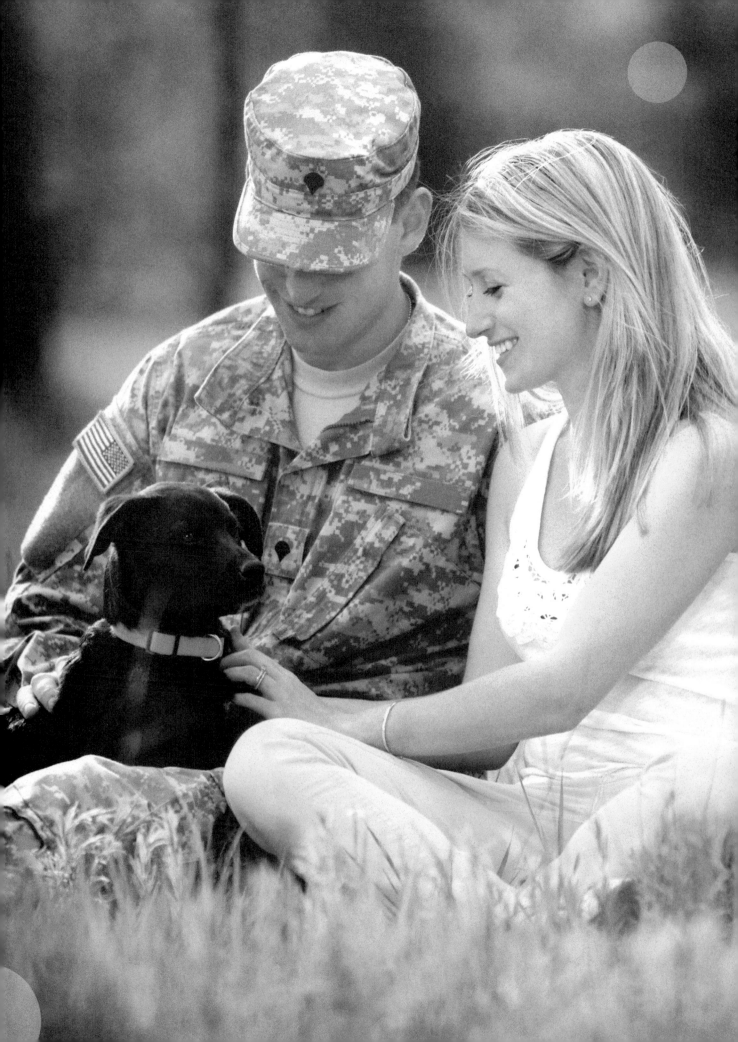

Lucky BUNNY

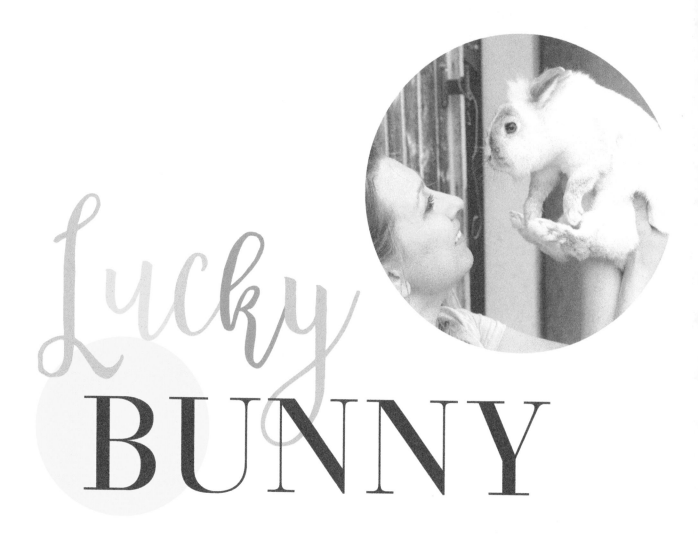

IT WAS A BEAUTIFUL, WARM JUNE EVENING AND I HAD JUST RETURNED home from a trip. I was pretty tired but forced myself to unpack and throw a load of laundry in before I hit the couch with my cats. After I finished these tasks, I laid down happily on the couch but was only there for a total of ten seconds when I realized I had forgotten to drag the garbage cans out to the curb for pickup the next morning. I really had to think whether I cared about the garbage pickup more than I cared about how good it felt to be lying down. After some serious contemplation, I reluctantly moved myself to walk outside and drag the bins across the acre of land to the end of the driveway and place them by the curb.

As I was trekking back up through the yard, I saw a black-and-white animal moving around in the tall grass. In the twilight, it was difficult to see if it was a small cat or a rabbit. Whatever it was, I thought to myself, it was probably missing from someone's home and if I could catch it, I could prevent it from being be eaten by a coyote that night—something that is a very real threat for domestic animals in my neck of the woods.

I walked slowly so I wouldn't startle the little creature, and as I got closer it looked to me like a fluffy little bunny. I blinked a few times to be sure, as it was getting darker quickly. It was definitely someone's missing family member. So I got down on my hands and knees and waited. I wanted the bunny to sense my energy—to see that I was soft, gentle, and not something to be afraid of. After a few minutes, I started to move toward him. I continued to quiet my energy by being conscious of my breathing and being patient. I sat near him in what had now become "our" space. He didn't run; he stayed. I sent him love from my heart to his. He continued to stay where he was, just hanging out, chewing on the grass. He would look at me now and then before returning his attention to chewing on the grass.

After a little while I said, "Bunny, you must let me save you or else you are going to be somebody's dinner tonight. It's not safe out here for you." I remained sitting and continued to breathe slowly as we sat in the silence together. I was with him and he was with me. When I held out my hand, the little bunny came right over to me and let me scoop him up in my arms. I wrapped him in inside my hoodie and we snuggled for a bit before I brought him inside.

I ended up posting about finding him on a local social media page and within hours his surprised, emotional, sweet little family came to get him. They were in shock that he had managed to survive for five days after their front gate had been mistakenly left open. It was definitely a happy ending to a situation that easily could have ended otherwise. I was so grateful that I had decided to take the garbage out that night! And that I had earned the trust of an animal. By slowing down,

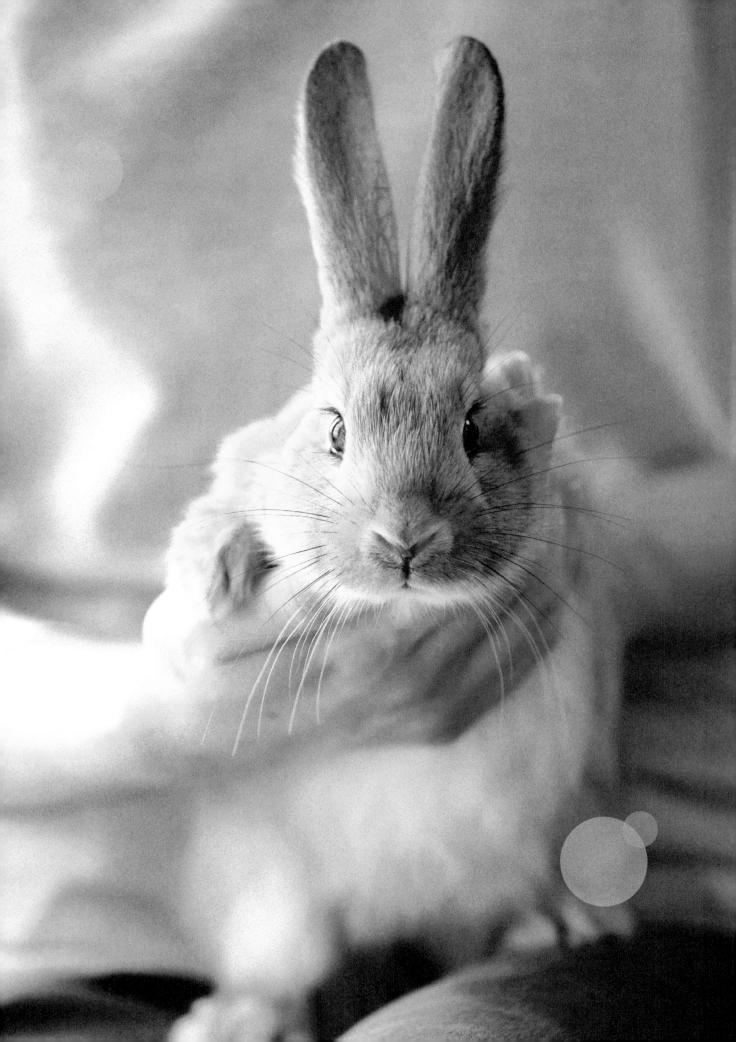

tuning in, and staying connected with his soul, I was able to extend my loving energy to show him he would be safe with me and I could help him. I was rewarded with his trust and he was rewarded with returning home to his family.

Distraction along with our natural inclination to move our bodies or minds can take away from the purity of a moment and the chance we have to be still.

Staying in the moment is not an easy thing to do. Our minds often race, thinking of a to-do list that awaits or someplace we're supposed to be. When you choose to stay even a moment longer, you can experience magic. This is true for traditional meditation or any of the other types of meditation I have described. An extra moment or even second can provide an insight that can change the dynamic of your relationship, open a door to new opportunities or activities, or just open your heart and provide you with a beautiful, memorable feeling to carry with you throughout the day or your life. A memory is a very powerful gift.

When you choose to stay even a moment longer, you can experience magic. An extra moment can provide an insight, open a door, or just open your heart.

Let me share with you now an experience I had when I chose to stay with a little bird. Because I chose to keep standing still (which was not easy!), it created an incredibly beautiful memory of love and trust for me that I will always cherish.

A Song
FOR ME

I WAS WORKING AT MY KITCHEN TABLE ONE MORNING WHEN I HEARD what sounded like a bird fly into the glass of the window beside me. Unfortunately for this little guy, that is exactly what happened. He landed, stunned and not moving in the thick leaves of bamboo shoots below the window. I ran outside to see if he was OK, and when I saw him lying there I picked him up and held him in my cupped hands, repeating "You are safe, you are loved, and everything is OK" while blowing warm air on his little body. I just sat with him hoping he would open his eyes. When he did, what happened next is something that I will carry with me always.

He didn't fly away. I told him that, when he felt ready, I would bring him back and find a nice branch for him to stand on and get his bearings. *He continued to stay with me.* I brought him over to the branch and lovingly tried to put his little feet on it, but he kept climbing back on to my finger! I gave up eventually and told him it was OK and that I understood he wasn't ready. I let him stay perched on my finger like a household pet and brought him close to my heart and kissed him on the head. *Still, he stayed with me.*

Next, this delicate little being climbed up on my shoulder and stood there. I turned my head to look at him and he just looked back at me. He proceeded to walk around to the back of my neck and play with my hair, and then he hopped back to my shoulder. My heart was so open, racing at the wonder of this experience. In that moment, the little bird started to sing a song into my ear and I clearly heard "thank you!" in his beautiful voice. We stood there in that magic for another minute or so and then I told him it was OK for him to go and I thanked him. Off he flew, to a branch above where I was standing. He sang for a few more moments and then flew away.

Being completely honest here, there were moments during this encounter when my excitement about what was happening

My heart was so open, racing at the wonder of this experience... the little bird started to sing a song into my ear

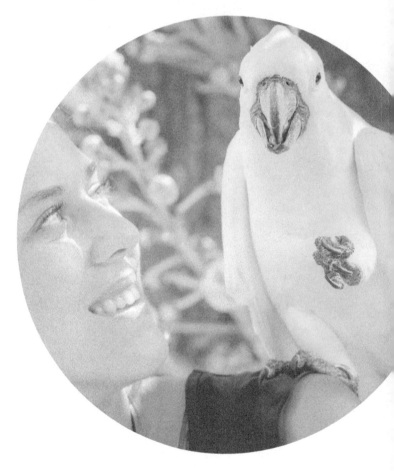

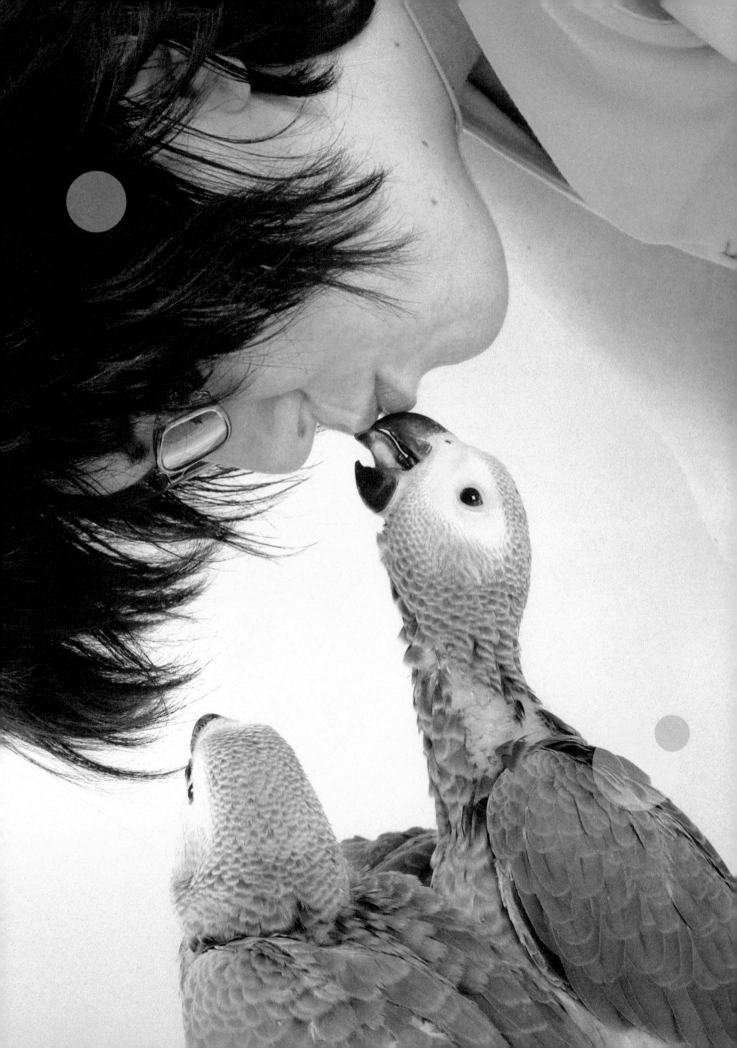

all nature is available to bring each of us back to ourselves

almost ruined it, and that was not what I wanted! I had to contain my energy, soften it, and bring it way down. I did this by breathing slowly to stay present and to calm and ground myself. The energy that had initially been excitement turned into a feeling of inner lightness and transcendence. It was a humming internal feeling, similar to what I have experienced in deep moments of meditation. The bird's continued presence and my desire to be with him fully and have him stay required this stillness. My reward was his acknowledgment that this energy was one that didn't trigger his instinct to flee; instead, it made him feel safe enough to stay. With our energies vibrating together in harmony, I felt united with nature on a cellular level and it was truly a natural high. He showed me that all nature is available to bring each of us back to ourselves if we allow it to; back to our beautiful soft spirits, where we are one with the world around us and within us.

The following meditation will assist you in becoming tuned in to yourself and the nature and animals around you in order to find moments of peace and stillness.

THE
Grow some roots
MEDITATION

I HAVE DONE THIS MEDITATION IN MANY DIFFERENT KINDS OF PLACES: at the barn while sitting in Tuxedo's stall with him, taking a seat under a shady tree with squirrels shuffling and darting around in the leaves nearby and birds in the trees above, and at home on my yoga mat after a wonderful practice with my cats on me or in the room, to name a few.

You want to start by tuning into the sounds of the beings that are around you. Let these sounds become the means of transport that carry you into their world. Once you feel a connection with this humming of nature, you can move to your breath.

- Take a deep breath in through your nose, feeling it flow down your throat, filling up your lungs and then your belly.

- Release that breath out of your mouth. Feel the breath you are releasing travel from your belly up through your lungs and throat and out of your mouth.

- Repeat this as many times as you like, enjoying the calm that comes from hearing your breathing.

- When you are ready, as you're breathing in and out, let go of anything you are holding on to. Anything that bothered you during the course of your day; anything that made you angry or upset sad, frustrated, stuck, or stressed.

- Put one hand on your heart and one hand on your belly. And as you breathe quietly, notice how comforting it feels to hold yourself. Stay with this for a few or as many breaths as feels good to you. Be fully with yourself first.

- Then, when you are ready, turn your full attention to this time with your own animal or the nature around you.

- Let your heart be open, making room for feelings of love, softness, gentleness, and kindness to surround you.

- At this point, I like to release all the tension I am holding in my shoulders and neck, and just let them drop down.

- Imagine you are a beautiful tree. Imagine the roots of that tree growing from beneath you, going deep down into the earth, making you strong and still.

- Imagine the branches of that tree growing out of you and reaching up to the sky in all directions. Visualize the connection below you and up above you. *Feel* the connection from below and above you.

- *Become* the tree.

- *Stay* in stillness.

Animals love when we stay in their presence and we are calm and still. We become a reflection of their natural state of chillness in the stillness.

Recycling ENERGY THROUGH THE ANIMAL METHOD

AS YOU'VE NOW LEARNED, THE ANIMAL METHOD ALLOWS YOU TO MOVE more mindfully through life with your animal companions, beginning by having an increased awareness of the present moment. It shines a light on your current inter-actions, patterns of behavior, and life situations, all of which transfer to and directly affect your animals. It's very important to be conscious of this fact. When we are stressed, out of balance, ill, or suffering, our animals take this on, and that energy can be reflected back on to us through their behavior or it can even manifest itself in illness in them. Conversely, when our animals are in need of something, they work hard to make us aware of the fact that they, too, have emotional, physical, and spiritual needs.

It is our responsibility to understand and find solutions to create harmony for our animals and for ourselves. The relationship is a continuous recycling of healing energy designed to give and take, thereby feeding both animal and guardian so that both can benefit from consistent support and unconditional love. The ancient Flower of Life symbol on the following page is likely one you have seen somewhere before, as it is a common image among artists, philosophers, architects, and many different spiritual and religious teachings all over the world. Its multiple overlapping circles make it a truly mesmerizing pattern that can draw you in as you meditate and can also serve as a beautiful reminder that a healthy relationship, whether it be with other people or our animal companions, benefits us at the highest level when loving energy is consistently being recycled. The interlacing of circles represents how we are all connected to each other, to nature, and to the universe.

The idea of interconnectedness can be found in the teachings of the Dalai Lama, who believes that our individual happiness is dependent on the happiness of others. In his book *Ethics for a New Millennium*, he claims that happiness does not come from purchasing and collecting material things but rather from a deep and genuine concern for the happiness of others. In fact, the Dalai

A healthy relationship benefits us at the highest level when loving energy is consistently being recycled.

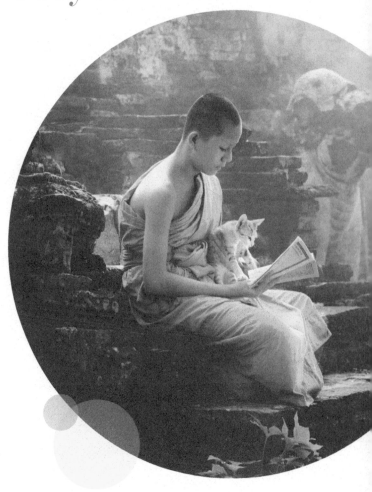

Flower of Life Symbol

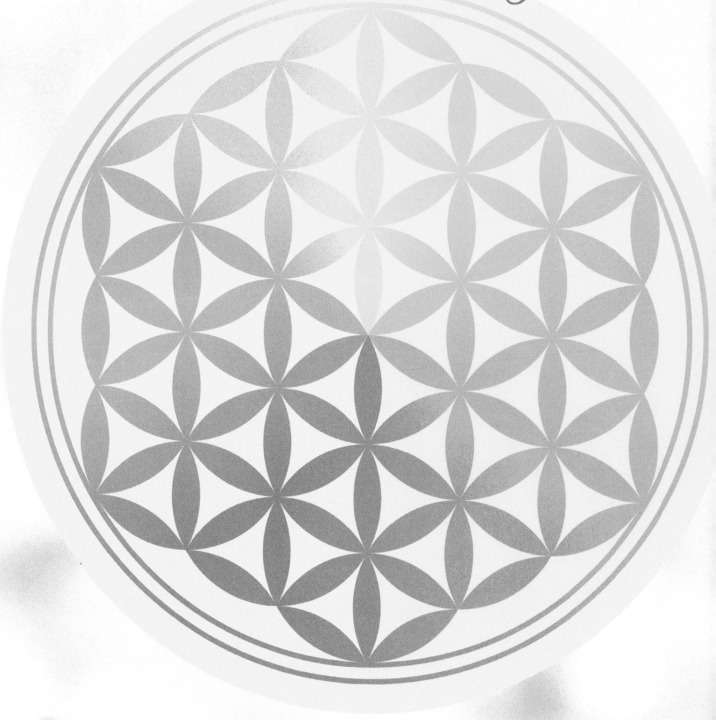

Lama contends that focusing on one's own needs instead of others' results in negative emotions that prevent true and lasting happiness for the self. Mahatma Gandhi held similar beliefs. One of my favorite quotes of his regarding self-understanding is, "The best way to find yourself is to lose yourself in the service of others." With this in mind, what better way to find yourself than through supporting those who live in service to you—the teachers, the healers right at your feet! Your animal companions!

Animals truly are the best teachers we could have for learning how to live mindfully and in the present moment. If you need further evidence of this fact, just consider your animals' natural state of being, and you will notice that they are doing The Animal Method with us:

- Our animals are in **AWE** of us! Think about how they react when we come home.

- Our animals **NOTICE** everything we do, think, and feel.

- Animals are **IN THE PRESENT MOMENT** at all times, which includes *our* present moment when we are together with them.

- An animal has a natural state of being similar to what we aspire to experience when we **MEDITATE**.

- Our animals **ALLOW** us to step out of our world and be with them in theirs.

- Our animals are an ultimate and endless source of unconditional **LOVE**.

- Our animals are able to **STAY** in stillness and peace, giving us the opportunity to join them.

I hope you and the animal companions in your life have fun exploring The Animal Method together, and that you reap all of the many benefits it has to offer. It has been my honor to share it with you!

the Animal
METHOD
—A WAY OF LIFE

NOT LONG AFTER I HAD FINISHED WRITING THIS BOOK, I HAD THE MOST profound experience, which came as a direct result of my own Meditating with Animals practice. Let me share it with you.

It started out as a regular day. I had gone to see Tuxedo and was planning to ride him in the arena; however, just as we were about to go inside, someone turned their horse out to run around for a bit, so I decided we'd go on a short trail ride and see if the arena was free when we returned. For what seemed like no particular reason to me, we went in a completely different direction than we normally go, winding up and down the hills randomly—or so I thought.

When we got to the top of this one hill, I asked Tux to go down the trail, but he refused to go in that direction, which is unusual as he is normally game to go anywhere. I sensed that he was agitated, so I changed my approach and asked him where he wanted to go, loosening the reins some more so he could be free to show me. He moved a few steps toward a flat, bushy area off the trail and I said with a laugh, "OK, we can go this way if you want to walk around that bush!" Off we went, but after just a few steps Tux stopped again, still agitated. I looked down and saw a light-blueish object lying in the dirt that looked like a chunk of cement or a piece of plastic. It was about the size of a tennis ball. Though it struck my curiosity, I initially dismissed it because I felt it probably wasn't worth the effort of jumping down and then having to get back up on Tux again. I tried to get him to move forward, but he seemed insistent that I get whatever that thing was down there. Realizing Tux wasn't going to give up, I said "OK!" and jumped off. I picked up the mysterious object. It fit in the palm of my hand and was heavy like a rock but unlike anything I'd ever seen. I stuffed it awkwardly and uncomfortably in the pocket of my riding pants and pulled Tuxedo up to an incline, where it was easier to hoist myself up onto his back. His energy was now noticeably different; he was totally calm and walked right back onto the trail without any resistance.

Later at home, I spent an hour searching the Internet to find out what kind of stone it was that I had picked up. I was amazed to discover that it is a masterpiece of nature: a botryoidal (meaning resembling the form of a bunch of grapes) blue agate or chalcedony.[32] Most astonishingly, I learned that the healing properties of this stone is that used to enhance one's

It felt as if I'd reunited with a long-lost friend or a piece of myself. Such a precious gift, and it's no coincidence that it was Tuxedo who led me to it.

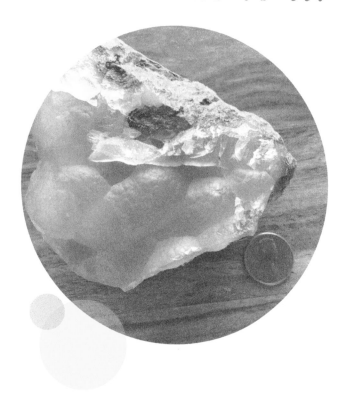

ability to communicate and is associated with the throat chakra. The voice of the body. I immediately connected the fact of having temporarily lost my voice when my vocal cord had been paralyzed from the removal of the cancerous thyroid tumor. But as I had slowly come to realize post-surgery, I had lost or given away my voice long before getting cancer, which I believe has a lot to do with why it happened. It is part of my journey in this life to have found my own voice again; to remember that I have one; and to not be afraid to speak my truth. And this personal growth is in large part thanks to the animal healers I had around me, as well as the divine timing of my life circumstances.

I can't explain how it felt to hold this stone that had such great personal significance—I didn't want to put it down. It felt as if I'd reunited with a long-lost friend or a piece of myself. Such a precious gift, and it's no coincidence that it was Tuxedo who led me to it. My magnificent, magical horse. And I soon discovered this special stone held even more significance for me.

I had first written about this experience in a blog post, and the day after I posted it I received an urging, an insistence, from my higher self, encouraging me to look up a photo of the thyroid gland. When I did I was blown away by what I saw: the thyroid gland looks *almost exactly* like my stone! The shape of the blue stone and its bubbly contours bear such a close resemblance to the gland, it is unbelievable. As I said, the stone made me feel like I found a piece of myself, and now this idea resonated even more deeply with me because it was my thyroid gland that had been removed when I was fighting cancer.

Having made this final realization, I was overcome with emotion, relief, and gratitude. I cried, releasing the remaining sadness and loss that had lingered from going through the frightening experience of being faced with my own mortality, realizing I had put those emotions aside in order to get through it. The following morning, I woke up feeling healed and whole with an even stronger appreciation for my precious animals and the power of Meditating with Animals. I recognized that there was no way I would have found the stone—and therefore my "missing piece"—otherwise. That day riding with Tux on the trails I was doing what I described in chapter 4 as the "Everything but the Kitchen Sink" meditation, which can involve walking, riding, singing, or any number of other activities.

Whatever it is you are doing with your animal, the key is to be present 100 percent. Because I was present with Tuxedo completely that day, he was able to guide me to this stone that holds such deep meaning for me. It has allowed me to see that nothing is ever permanently lost and that energy is transformed. It reminds me that I have a voice and I can choose how I want it to be heard.

Our animals are our spirit guides. Their wisdom is beyond what we can ever know or understand on our own. This is why, if we take the time to just *be* with them, a world of new experiences, even magic, can be open to us.

Acknowledgments

THANK YOU TO THE SPECIAL ANIMAL SOULS THAT ARE NOW A PART OF mine: Duke, Duchess, Thomas, Kitty, Heidi, Red, Sammy, Bailey, Tripp, Honey, Ruby, Thomas 2, Mr. A, Mommy Cat, Sophie, Striped Cat, Black Dog, Sylvester, Beauty School, Kit-Ten, Shark, and Tuxedo, my love.

I would also like to thank my amazing friends and family and the powerful goddess women warriors and spiritual teachers who supported me and lifted me up with their presence, love, and guidance. All of you helped me weather the wild, powerful, and seemingly endless storm that life threw my way. I know it wasn't easy and it did take a village. I love you and am full of gratitude for each of you:

Friends: Andy, Lisa, Victoria, Laurie, Joyce, Heidi, and Lawrence

Family: Mom, Grandma (in spirit), Kathy, Ben, Adriane, and Aunt Carol

Powerful goddess women warriors and spiritual teachers:

Kelly, Andrea, Suzan, and Zhena

I give special thanks to Zhena Muzyka for her encouragement, inspiration, and guidance in showing me I had a book inside me waiting to be released to the world. It was through our work together that *Meditating with Animals* was brought to life.

I extend my deepest gratitude to Dr. Lois Barnes, MD, for being the angel who found my cancer. You were put in my life in perfect divine timing and are the reason I am here now writing this book.

I give additional thanks to Dr. Robert Ruder, my awesome surgeon, for your thorough diagnosis, skilled care, and genuine kindness during a difficult time, and to Dr. Tricia Westhoff Pankratz (Dr. W) for your knowledgeable aftercare and being super cool and patient with me when I know I must have been really annoying.

I would also like to thank my father for being who he was because he made me who I AM.

Thank you to Emily Dickinson for these beautiful words that I have always felt were written for me:

If I can stop one heart from breaking,
I shall not live in vain.
If I can ease one life the aching,
Or cool one pain,
Or help one fainting robin
Unto his nest again,
I shall not live in vain.

With all the love in my heart,
—Pamela

About the
AUTHOR

PAMELA ROBINS IS A PASSIONATE AND ENTHUSIASTIC STUDENT OF continuous learning and personal growth through traditional therapy, intuitive studies and guidance, healing work, and nature. She has been driven to take on many roles throughout her life, including that of entrepreneur, inspirational guide, and now author.

One of her entrepreneurial endeavors involved designing and creating specialty home decor items, which were sold worldwide and featured in the Philadelphia Museum of Art, the *New York Times* Style section, and various fashion magazines, in addition to being selected for the set of *Friends* and MTV's *The Real World*. Pamela also created and designed her own equestrian apparel line. Called Horseworship, it features fine art photography and her own original poetry and is sold to horse lovers around the world.

Pamela is a competitive equestrian in the sport of three-day eventing; a yoga, meditation, Reiki, and singing bowl practitioner; and a fitness enthusiast. She enjoys inspiring others and living a healthy lifestyle in California with her two incredible cats, Sylvester and Kit-Ten, and her horse, Tuxedo.

For more information about The Animal Method™ or to book a private session with Pamela, please visit www.meditatingwithanimals.com.

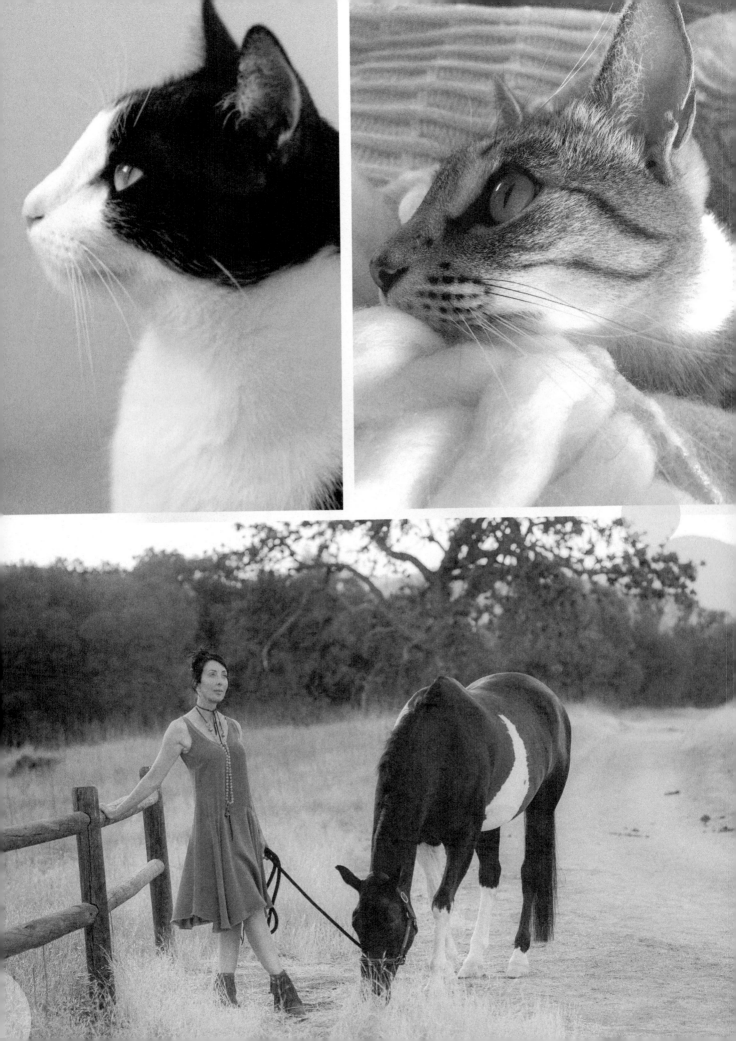

ENDNOTES

1. Bekoff, Marc PhD. "Do Animals Have Spiritual Experiences? Yes they do." *Psychology Today* (November 2009)

2. Viegas, Jennifer. "Animals said to have Spiritual Experiences." Discovery News/NBCnews.com (October 2010)

3. Keltner, Dacher. "Awe: For Altruism and Health?" Slate.com, John Templeton Foundation (n.d.)

4. Makin, Simon. "Feeling Awe may be good for our health." Scientificamerican.com (Sept. 2015)

5. Hirst, K. Kris. "Archeology Expert." About.com (2016)

6. Palermo, Elizabeth. "Why Do Cats Bring Home Dead Animals?" Livescience.com (March 2013)

7. Humanesociety.org. "Cat Chat: Understanding Feline Language."

8. Grieves, Deidre. "Tamar Geller Shares 5 Fascinating Behaviors Dogs Inherit From Wolves." Pet360.com

9. Woofpedia.com (by The American Kennel Club). "Why Does My Dog Kick Her Back Legs Over Her Poop?"

10. Lyons, Leslie A. "Why Do Cats Purr?" Scientificamerican.com (April 2006)

11. Steinberg, Rebecca M. "Sense Organs." *Animal Sciences* (September 2002)

12. Griffin, Ashley. "Horse Hearing." University of Minnesota (Extension) (2015)

13. Ghose, Tia. "Feline Vision: How Cats See the World." *Live Science* (2013)

14. Tyson, Peter. "Dogs' Dazzling Sense of Smell." *Nova* (2012)

15. Braun, David Maxwell. "The Health and Emotional Benefits of human-animal interaction." Nationalgeographic.com (September 2009)

16. Castillo, Michelle. "Americans Will Spend More Than $60 Billion On Their Pets This Year." NBCnews.com (July 2015)

17. "Meditation...Towards A Stress Free Life." Healthandyoga.com

18. Walia, Arjun. "It Works: New Study Outlines What Meditation, Yoga and Prayer Can Do To The Human Body." Collective-Evolution.com (January 2016)

19. McGreevey, Sue. "Eight Weeks to a Better Brain." *Harvard Gazette* (January 2011)

20. McCraty, Rollin PhD, Atkinson, Mike, Tomasino, Dana, B.A., and Tiller, William A. PhD. "The Electricity of Touch: Detection and Measurement of Cardiac Energy Exchange Between People." HeartMath Institute. Heartmath.org (1998)

21. Weil, Andrew, MD. "Breathing: Three Exercises." Drweil.com

22. Porterfield, Traci. "5 Ways to Become a Magnet for Love." The Chopra Center, Chopra.com (2016)

23. Wagner, Susan DVM, MS, DACVIM. "The Energy of the Human-Animal Bond." DVM.360

24. Ibid.

25. Dosa, M. David MD, MPH. "A Day in the Life of Oscar the Cat." *The New England Journal of Medicine* (July 2007)

26. Reporter, *Daily Mail*. "The greatest love of all: Study shows why humans are capable of caring unconditionally." Dailymail.com (April 2009)

27. Nodiff-Netanel, Victoria, Minitherapyhorses.com

28. Becker, Marty, Dr. "Dr. Marty Becker: The Healing Power of Pets." Purina.com (September 2015)

29. Clores, Suzanne. "The Benefits of Quiet for Body, Mind and Spirit." Nextavenue.org (February 2012)

30. Ibid.

31. Tolle, Eckhart. *Stillness Speaks*. New World Library: Novato, CA (2003). Accessed at soulfulliving.com

32. "Blue Chalcedony," HealingCrystals.com

RESOURCES

www.apexprotectionproject.org

www.bitchfix.com

www.blackjaguarwhitetiger.org

www.canterusa.org

www.cawildlife.org

www.cocosanimalwelfare.org

www.davidshepherd.org
(Elephant Orphanage Project)

www.farmsanctuary.org

www.gamerangersinternational.org

www.gentlebarn.org

www.guidedog.org

www.heartmath.org

www.horseworship.com

www.janegoodall.org

www.malibuvets.com

www.mercyforanimals.org

www.minitherapyhorses.com

www.peta.org

www.returntofreedom.org

www.searchdogfoundation.org

www.seashepherd.org

www.tereraitrent.org

www.theloveddog.com

www.thoughtgenius.com

www.tikkihywoodtrust.org

www.wingsofrescue.org

www.zhena.tv

Instagram: @dr_shawa_vet

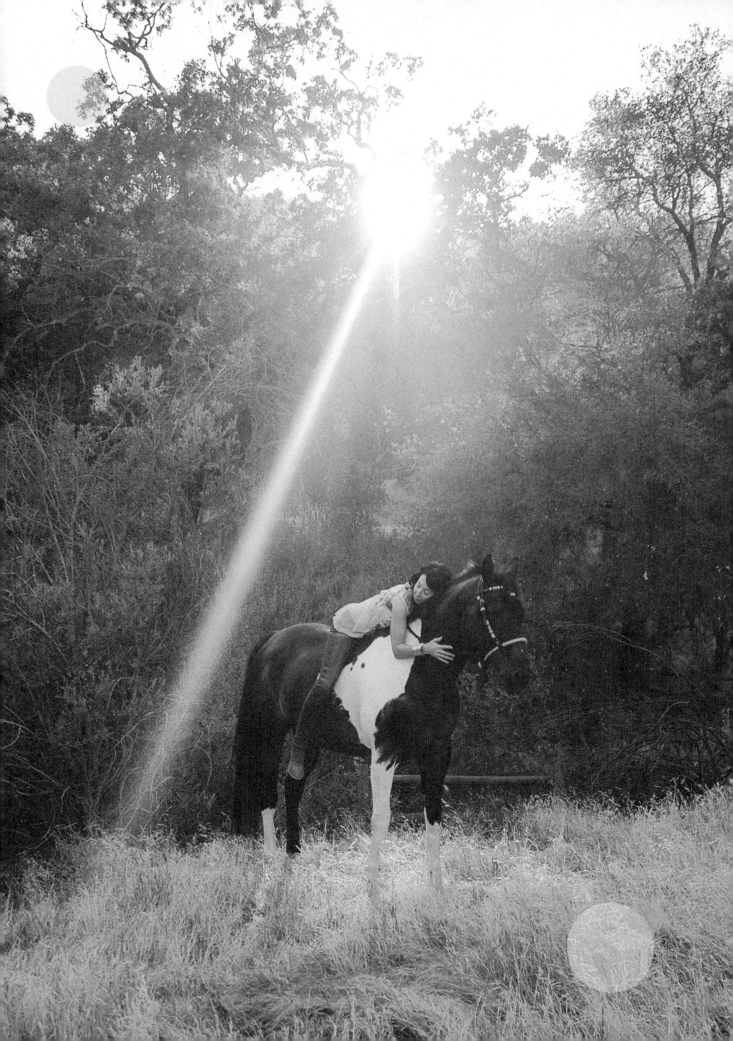

CPSIA information can be obtained
at www.ICGtesting.com
Printed in the USA
FSOW04n1724261116
27739FS